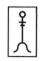

Also by Will Wilkoff, M.D.

COPING WITH A PICKY EATER

IS MY CHILD OVERTIRED?

WILL WILKOFF, M.D.

The Maternity Leave Breastfeeding Plan

HOW TO ENJOY NURSING FOR THREE
MONTHS AND GO BACK TO WORK GUILT-FREE

A Fireside Book
Published by Simon & Schuster

New York   London   Toronto   Sydney   Singapore

This publication contains the opinions and ideas of its author. It is intended to provide helpful and informative material on the subjects addressed in the publication. It is sold with the understanding that the author and publisher are not engaged in rendering medical, health, or any other kind of personal professional services in the book. The reader should consult his or her medical, health, or other competent professional before adopting any of the suggestions in this book or drawing inferences from it.

The author and publisher specifically disclaim all responsibility for any liability, loss, or risk, personal or otherwise, which is incurred as a consequence, directly or indirectly, of the use and application of any of the contents of this book.

FIRESIDE
Rockefeller Center
1230 Avenue of the Americas
New York, NY 10020

Copyright © 2002 by William Wilkoff, M.D.
All rights reserved, including the right of reproduction
in whole or in part in any form.

FIRESIDE and colophon are registered trademarks
of Simon & Schuster, Inc.

For information about special discounts for bulk purchases,
please contact Simon & Schuster Special Sales:
1-800-456-6789 or business@simonandschuster.com

Designed by Lauren Simonetti
Manufactured in the United States of America
10 9 8 7 6 5 4 3 2 1

Library of Congress Cataloging-in-Publication Data
Wilkoff, William G.
The maternity leave breastfeeding plan : how to enjoy nursing for three months
and go back to work guilt-free / Will Wilkoff
p. cm.
Includes index.
1. Breast feeding. 2. Maternity leave. I. Title.
RJ216.W675 2002
649'.33—dc21   2002021044
ISBN 0-7432-1345-9

To
Jenn, Em, and Nick

Acknowledgments

I would like to thank the thousands of parents here on the coast of Maine who have permitted me to participate in the care of their children. They have continued to ask my advice even though they know I don't always have the right answers. They still give me undeserved credit for good suggestions that they suspect I have borrowed from other, more experienced parents. Although they know where I live and can find my number in the telephone book, they have allowed me to enjoy my days off without interruption.

My associates, Dr. Deborah Hagler and Dr. Andrea Loeffler, provide such competent and compassionate care to my patients when they are on call that I wonder why any parent bothers to request an appointment with me. Their arrival in Brunswick has allowed me to repay the sleep debt that I accumulated over my first twenty years in practice. Without them I would never have found the time to write this book.

My mother taught me to value common sense, but it is my wife, Marilyn, who has encouraged me to become a better listener. I thank her for being my harshest critic, moral compass, and best friend for the last thirty-four years.

CONTENTS

CONTENTS

The
Maternity Leave
Breastfeeding
Plan

I

Do We Really Need Another Book About Breastfeeding?

It doesn't make much sense. Nursing an infant would appear to be such a simple biologic process. We seem to get along just fine without detailed instructions on how to perform our other "natural" body functions. However, "experts" continue to write books about breastfeeding. Amazon.com already lists more than two hundred titles that offer advice about nursing. How could there possibly be anything new to say about breastfeeding babies?

After all, humans have been nursing their offspring for tens of thousands of years. Why do we need another self-proclaimed expert to tell us how to do it? Particularly if that "expert" doesn't even have breasts himself.

There are numerous reasons why we need a fresh perspective on breastfeeding. First, despite the efforts of physician groups such as the American Academy of Pediatrics; public health officials, including the Surgeon General; and other breastfeeding advocacy organizations, we have made little, if any, progress in encouraging women to nurse their newborn infants. Only about 60 to 65 percent of new mothers decide to breastfeed. Of those women a good many stop nursing before their babies are a month old. By the time they are six months old, 20 percent of all babies are still being breastfed; among babies whose mothers have returned to work, only 10 percent of all babies are still breastfed. Our society is doing a poor job of recruiting women to breastfeed and is doing little or nothing to create an environment that will support those mothers who decide to nurse their babies. In the nearly thirty years that I have been practicing pediatrics, these statistics have not changed significantly.

Many mothers who have managed to nurse longer than a few weeks have told me that they have found breastfeeding confining, tiring, and unsatisfying. Although they may plan to nurse their next child, these women see this as a decision to make a sacrifice for the good of their babies. The mothers who abandon their nursing plan frequently feel that they have failed at their first attempt at parenting.

The bottom line is that we continue to do a poor job of promoting what most scientists agree is the best first food for infants. The books that have been written about breastfeeding, while factually accurate, have somehow missed the mark. We do an even worse job of educating and supporting those women who do accept the challenge, and when they don't succeed, we make them feel like failures.

Over the last quarter century of practicing pediatrics in a small college town on the coast of Maine, I have had ample opportunity to experience this sad state of affairs firsthand. I have attempted to encourage mothers to nurse when I speak at childbirth classes. I offer as much advice and emotional support as I can to the women who decide to breastfeed. Although a recent survey of breastfeeding in our community suggests that my patients are being nursed longer than those in other pediatric practices, I continue to encounter mothers who have stopped breastfeeding prematurely. Many of them have tearfully shared with me their frustration and disappointment.

Frustrated myself by the fact that too few women are choosing to breastfeed and saddened by the fact that many who do nurse aren't enjoying it, I decided to see if there was something more I could do to improve the situation. First, I had to consider the reasons for our poor success rate. Although the anatomy and physiology of the human breast has not changed in thousands of years, the demands on women have changed dramatically. When we were hunter-gatherers roaming the African savanna, mothers and their infants were in constant contact. Babies could breastfeed at will while mates and clan members were available to protect and nurture the vulnerable nursing mothers. Even as recently as a century ago the majority of women were at home with their children. Although they shouldered the majority of the household chores, mothers still had the time to breastfeed. Inexperienced mothers also had easy access to their mothers and older sisters who could function as knowledgeable breastfeeding advisers.

Compare that to the situation at the beginning of the twenty-first century. In 1970 less than 40 percent of women with children worked, but today 55 percent of child-bearing women will return to a job when their maternity leaves end. Today's new mothers may not have been breastfed themselves, and even if they were, the baby's grandmother may live too far away to serve as a hands-on adviser for more than just a few days. When a new mother does return to work, she and her baby will be together for slightly more than half of each day, and more than 50 percent of that time both will be (or at least should be) sleeping. This whole process doesn't sound so "natural" anymore, does it? It won't be surprising if breastfeeding doesn't come naturally.

This mismatch between the biologic demands of nursing and the lifestyle of the average working mother wasn't the only discrepancy I discovered as I continued my search for answers. I realized that the way we were promoting breastfeeding was actually discouraging some women from nursing. For example, the American Academy of Pediatrics has told parents that "exclusive breastfeeding is ideal nutrition" for the first six months and suggested that "breastfeeding continue for at least twelve months." Obviously the academy didn't intend to discourage women, but six months can sound unrealistic to a mother whose maternity leave is over in three.

In their attempt to promote what they know is the best way to feed babies, other breastfeeding advocacy groups are perceived as militant zealots who are willing to nurse their infants and young children anywhere, anytime, and to solve any problem. It isn't surprising that women who know they will be returning to jobs in twelve weeks are intimidated, discouraged, or just plain turned off by advice from sources that apparently don't understand an individual's situation or preferences. In other words, by overemphasizing the commitment that breastfeeding requires we have discouraged many working women from nursing, *and* we have made others feel guilty when they can't meet those unreasonable expectations.

No question about it, breastfeeding does require a bigger commitment than formula feeding during the first week or two when a new mother's body is adjusting to its role as a nutritional source. However, women don't have to nurse for a year or even six months to provide their babies with many, if not most, of the benefits of breastfeeding. Isn't there some way that we could get this message out and promote breastfeeding realistically in a style that would make sense for, and appeal to, working mothers?

As I looked for more answers, I discovered an interesting research paper written by two nurse-educators. These researchers observed that the working mothers in their study group who had planned shorter breastfeeding durations reported higher satisfaction with breastfeeding while still meeting the demands of their professional roles. I had noticed the same phenomenon myself. Maybe we could help more working mothers enjoy rewarding nursing experiences by advocating a shorter, more realistic breastfeeding plan. Focusing our promotional and educational efforts on this achievable goal of breastfeeding for the first three months, the length of a typical maternity leave in the United States, was the obvious choice.

As I thought more about why women stopped breastfeeding, I remembered the tearful voices of nursing mothers who had told me how tired they were and how tied down they felt. In fact during my research I discovered several studies by other physicians and nurses that listed maternal fatigue as the primary reason that mothers stopped breastfeeding. However, I know plenty of nursing mothers who haven't complained about being exhausted or confined by nursing. What was different about their experiences? The answer was that these women had not allowed themselves to become their babies' pacifiers. These mothers, sometimes by good luck, sometimes with my assistance, had helped their infants learn to put themselves to sleep. By separating breastfeeding from the sleep process, these women were able to nurse longer and enjoy the experience while those women who had allowed their breasts to become pacifiers were becoming sleep-deprived zombies. Doesn't it make sense to incorporate good sleep management strategies into our breastfeeding education programs?

It also occurred to me that the majority of women who stop nursing prematurely do so in the first few weeks. The first ten to fourteen days can be filled with anxiety, uncertainty, confusion, and discomfort. Nursing mothers who can ride out this stormy period without switching their babies to formula are very likely to continue breastfeeding until they return to work. Most mothers begin their breastfeeding experience in a hospital, though, unfortunately, many hospitals lack enough trained staff to help nursing mothers get a good start. In fact, many hospitals have policies that unintentionally discourage breastfeeding. Only a handful of hospitals in this country have even attempted to become certified as "Baby-Friendly" by WHO (the World Health Organization). Even fewer have been awarded this certification that recognizes hospitals with policies and practices that promote breastfeeding. If we want to help more women succeed at breastfeeding, we had better sharpen our focus on those critical two weeks immediately after the baby is born.

After mulling over these and other reasons for our disappointing breastfeeding record, I was ready to think about what we could do about it. First came the realization that I needed to scrap the "we" concept. Although I am a card-carrying member of the American Academy of Pediatrics, I am certainly not a "joiner" by nature, nor am I a person with much political savvy or influence. I also knew that the approach to breastfeeding that was beginning to crystallize in my mind was going to be too radical to be promptly embraced by most traditional breastfeeding advocates.

Although, swift, decisive, and substantive action by the executive and/or legislative branches of the federal government could create an economic environment that would encourage more working women to breastfeed, something told me that wasn't going to happen. If a Democratic administration that had been talking about the plight of the working woman for eight years couldn't get it done, there seemed little hope that any progress would be made during subsequent administrations.

A few enlightened corporations have created personnel policies that promote breastfeeding (only 7 percent provide designated rooms for pumping), but I didn't see much evidence that the example they set was going to trigger a national trend. It was beginning to look as though if I wanted to help working women fit breastfeeding into their lives, I was going to have to act on my own. I had already written a couple of books for parents that had been reasonably well received. If only I could convince a publisher that I had something new to say about breastfeeding. Fortunately the people at Simon & Schuster realized quickly that there was room on the shelves for yet another book about breastfeeding, and so *The Maternity Leave Breastfeeding Plan* was written. I will promise you as I promised them, this book really is different. If you are a working woman, it can help you enjoy a successful and rewarding breastfeeding experience.

2

What Is the Maternity Leave Breastfeeding Plan?

The Maternity Leave Breastfeeding Plan is a collection of strategies that will allow you and your baby to enjoy the advantages of breastfeeding until your maternity leave has ended. It acknowledges that because the combination of breastfeeding and even part-time employment can be difficult, you may have no other option than to wean your baby after three months, when it is time to go back to work. The Plan will help you understand that although weaning before your baby wants to stop nursing may be a sad time, it need not be a guilt-fest or a reason to abandon breastfeeding before you have even begun.

Three months of nursing will give you and your baby an excellent start as parent and child. However, if you decide to continue nursing when your maternity leave is over, *The Maternity Leave Breastfeeding Plan* includes strategies that will significantly improve your chances of mastering the challenge.

At the heart of *The Maternity Leave Breastfeeding Plan* is the observation that maternal fatigue is one of the most important reasons, if not the most important reason, that women stop breastfeeding. A good portion of the book in your hands is aimed at keeping you well rested by recruiting a competent and empathetic support group, trimming your schedule and responsibilities, and, most important, avoiding the role of pacifier.

Because the first two weeks of nursing are usually the most difficult, *The Maternity Leave Breastfeeding Plan* focuses on this critical period with time-tested advice about such topics as the first nursing, attachment problems, engorgement, and nipple soreness. To help you endure what can seem like an interminable wait until your milk comes in, the Plan reassures you and tells how to forge a working relationship with your pediatrician so you won't have to worry that your baby will become undernourished while you wait.

Once nursing is well established the Plan shows you how to balance breastfeeding with your other responsibilities and interests. Nursing does require a commitment, but mothers who follow the Maternity Leave Breastfeeding Plan won't feel that nursing has taken over their lives. In other words, this is a mother-friendly approach to nursing.

While most books about breastfeeding give little attention to the topic of weaning, when it is time to stop breastfeeding, the Plan will walk you through the process, step by step. With support and encouragement, this often difficult transition can be achieved with minimal emotional trauma to you and your baby.

In summary, the Maternity Leave Breastfeeding Plan is a realistic, mother-friendly, commonsense approach to nursing that can allow a working mother and her infant to enjoy the benefits of breastfeeding and help them prepare for either weaning or continued breastfeeding when the maternity leave is over.

3

WHY SHOULD I BREASTFEED MY BABY?

Because you want to! You already know that breastfeeding isn't always easy. If you hope to nourish your baby with only breast-milk for the first three months, or if you accept the bigger challenge of continuing to nurse after you go back to your "paying job," you must be committed. Breastfeeding must be something that you want to do, or it just won't work. For example, if you are nursing your baby only because someone else (i.e., your doctor, partner, mother, or sister) thinks it is important, you are much more likely to reach for a bottle of formula when your nipples become cracked and painful.

Although I hope to convince as many women as I can to breastfeed their babies for the first three months, I don't want you to nurse your baby merely because "Dr. Wilkoff says it's the right thing to do." Nor do I want you to breastfeed because your younger sister did. Raising children is not a competitive sport, and nursing your baby for two months longer than your sister did won't show your parents or anyone else that you're a better woman.

Breastfeeding is not about pleasing your husband or your obstetrician. Nursing is simply the most natural way to feed your baby, but it also should be a positive experience for *you*. If you are doing it to meet someone else's expectations, you are setting yourself up for an unpleasant double disappointment should you decide to stop before "they" think it is time.

Breastfeeding is not the only way to nourish your baby. You do have a choice. I hope that when you have finished reading *The Maternity Leave Breastfeeding Plan,* you will realize that some of the negative things you have heard about breastfeeding either aren't true or can be avoided with the strategies I have suggested. You don't have to breastfeed for a whole year or even six months for you and your child to benefit from the experience. Nor do you have to breastfeed in public if it makes you uncomfortable. In other words, I want you to understand that nursing need not require the "total" commitment that you may have been hesitant or unwilling to make. Breastfeeding does, however, require one important commitment. You must *want* to breastfeed. If your motivation comes from within, it will be there to support you when the going gets tough. On the other hand, if breastfeeding is someone else's idea, you may well abandon the effort during the first long and sleepless night.

I trust that after reading this book you will not only decide that nursing is something you *want* to do, but also something you *can* do in a way that makes you feel good about yourself. If I have failed to convince you that breastfeeding is worth the effort, then it is my failure and not yours. I will be content knowing that you have at least thought about the pros and cons and decided it isn't something you want to do. I am not interested in arm twisting or sending you on a guilt trip. It is more important for me to know that you are comfortable being a parent, regardless of whether you breastfeed or not.

It's the natural thing to do. Over the last thirty years I have read and listened to scores of experts expound on the benefits of breastfeeding. For the most part I have been disappointed that so few of them have been able to produce dramatic statistics to support the often quoted assertion that "breast is best." While the results of each individual study may not offer impressive evidence, when taken as a whole, the research on breastfeeding does provide us with ample evidence of its superiority. And with each year more studies are published that demonstrate new and unexpected benefits of breastfeeding.

I am not much of a numbers person. Even well-intentioned scientists often report and misinterpret data that they find themselves retracting a few years later. The bottom line is that while I am reassured by the research that supports breastfeeding, I recommend breastfeeding to my patients because *it's the natural thing to do*, not because of what I have read in any book or medical journal.

Why would you be put on this earth with two breasts that make milk, if that milk wasn't the best thing to feed your baby? Scientists are never going to discover all of its benefits because human milk is a very complex substance that has evolved over millions of years to meet the particular needs of our species. For example, we know that seals provide their pups with milk that is extremely high in calories and rich in fat. This nutritional composition is important for their survival in the frigid ocean waters in which they live. It just makes sense that your milk must contain a mixture of nutritional ingredients and disease-preventing elements uniquely suited to the needs of your infant.

Formula companies brew up products using cow's milk or soy protein that allows human babies to grow at a rate that is similar to infants who are nursed by their mothers. However, not even the scientists who have devised the formulas claim that they have created a substance that contains all of the beneficial elements breastmilk contains.

IF YOU WANT MORE REASONS TO BREASTFEED YOUR BABY

There isn't enough space in this little book to comment on all of the benefits that have been claimed for breastfeeding. Therefore, I have chosen to present only a few of the most well-publicized claims. In some cases there may not be enough consistent data to substantiate a claim, but I have included it because I think it is important that you aren't the victim of unrealistic expectations.

Remember, the best reason to nurse your baby is because it is the natural thing to do. Just because we can't prove that your child will be smarter or run faster because he is breastfed doesn't mean that you should second-guess your decision to nurse.

Research about breastfeeding is very difficult to interpret because there are so many factors that must be considered. How old were the mothers? Was their culture similar to ours? What was their economic situation? Did the children attend daycare? How long did the babies breastfeed and was formula offered as a supplement? When were solid foods introduced? As you read the next few pages remember how questions like this could confuse the results of any one study.

Protection against infections. We know that breast milk, particularly colostrum (the first substance that your breasts produce) is rich in antibodies and other infection-preventing substances. However, we have relatively little information about the specific nature and effectiveness of these ingredients.

In underdeveloped countries where water supplies may be unsafe and sanitation facilities are often nonexistent, the benefit of breastfeeding is easy to demonstrate. It is not surprising that babies who are given formula mixed with water that may be contaminated have more infections than babies who are drinking breastmilk that contains protective antibodies.

In more highly developed societies, such as ours in North America, it has been more difficult to demonstrate the benefits of breastfeeding. Safe water systems, sophisticated sanitation systems, immunizations, and antibiotics have reduced the risk of infection to a level that makes the advantages of nursing more difficult to detect. However, there is some consistent evidence that breastfed infants have fewer **ear infections.** Of course this is not complete protection, and one researcher's data suggests that breastfeeding only helps reduce the risk of the initial infection and not recurrences. There are other factors that appear to be more closely linked to the development of ear infections—exposure to cigarette smoke and daycare are the two most obvious.

Lower respiratory illnesses such as bronchitis, bronchiolitis, and pneumonia may be less likely to occur among babies who are breastfed. Unfortunately exposure to large numbers of small children in a confined area (i.e., daycare) and respiratory irritants such as cigarette smoke and air pollution seem to cancel out or overwhelm this benefit of nursing.

Diarrheal illnesses may also occur less frequently in breastfed babies. This has been clearly demonstrated for the bacteria Salmonella, but is probably also true for viral gastroenteritis, which is much more common. In my personal experience, I have noticed that breastfed babies seem to get over their gastrointestinal illnesses more quickly than their bottlefed counterparts.

Some very recent research suggests that **urinary tract infections** are less likely to develop in breastfed infants. This is probably the result of the fact that nursing children have less harmful bacteria in their intestines, and not because of antibodies present in the milk.

Many of these studies are very preliminary and the benefits are not dramatic. Some breastfeeding mothers are surprised when their infant gets a cold or develops an ear infection because someone had led them to believe that by nursing they were providing their baby with excellent protection against infection. Remember, breastfeeding offers only *some* protection. Handwashing and avoiding cigarette smoke and groups of small children are at least as important in protecting your infant from infection.

Protection against other diseases. Some epidemiological studies have suggested that breastfed babies are less likely to develop juvenile-onset diabetes and some digestive disorders including Crohn's disease and lymphoma (a form of cancer). It is suspected that this may be related to immunological components or anti-inflammatory properties of breastmilk. Again, I must warn you that these observations are purely statistical. They may not stand up to the test of time and are merely something to keep in mind.

Delaying the onset of allergic symptoms. It was once believed that human breasts acted as filters protecting your baby from allergens in your diet. Some physicians hoped that by delaying the exposure to allergens (i.e., by breastfeeding) until your child was older that allergic symptoms would be less likely to develop. Unfortunately, the story doesn't seem to be that simple and the evidence supporting this theory is controversial.

Your child is exposed to allergens in many different ways, not just through what she eats. The air she breathes and the substances that touch her skin all may contain material that can trigger an allergic reaction. However, because there is some evidence that suggests that breastfeeding may delay, but probably not prevent, your child from developing allergic symptoms, I strongly suggest that you start by nursing your baby if you have a family history of asthma or eczema. Even if nursing only *delays* the onset of the symptoms until your child is older, this must be considered an advantage. There will be so many other challenges for you to master during your child's first year of life, that you don't want asthma or eczema to make your job of parenting any more difficult than it needs to be.

Nutritional advantages. You probably won't hear your pediatrician claim that your baby will grow bigger and faster if he is breastfed. She has noticed that her breastfed patients usually grow a bit slower initially and are often not as heavy as their bottlefed counterparts. This isn't necessarily a bad thing, and it doesn't mean that your child will end up being shorter than average because you nursed her.

Your breastmilk will contain a collection of nutrients that should be uniquely tailored to your child's needs. For example, the fat content of human milk varies depending on who the mother is and what she eats. Some women have more fat in their milk than others, and every woman can change the fat content of her milk by making drastic changes in the fat content of her diet.

I have reviewed one study that found that children who were breastfed had a more "favorable" lipoprotein profile (that is, cholesterol and the other body fats) than bottlefed babies. Another survey, done in Bavaria, demonstrated that on average children who were breastfed were less likely to be overweight when they started school. The bottom line is that there are nutritional advantages to breastmilk, but they are sometimes difficult to determine because we too often assume that bigger is better.

Intelligence. In the last few years there has been considerable debate and confusion about the importance of the first few years in the development of a child's intelligence. Some "experts" have claimed that the first three years represent a window of opportunity during which parents should expose their child to a stimulating environment that will maximize intellectual capacity. More recently, other "experts" have provided evidence that a child's genes may be more important in the ultimate determination of her intelligence, and that you don't have to worry about making sure that her every waking hour is filled with stimulating words and music. Breastfeeding has been swept up in the controversy as well. At least one study suggests that babies who are nursed end up with higher IQs than those who were bottlefed. However, the advantage appears to be extremely small and is counterbalanced by an observation in the same study that children who used pacifiers had lower IQs, whether they were breast- or bottle-fed.

I don't think I can say it any better than two Canadian pediatricians who observed, "The best evidence is that intelligent, loving and caring mothers are likely to have intelligent children, irrespective of how they choose to feed their babies."*

Reducing the risk of SIDS. There are some statistics which suggest that infants who are being breastfed are less likely to die without explanation. Although we frequently attribute these deaths to Sudden Infant Death Syndrome (SIDS), they are certainly not due to a single disease or condition. SIDS is merely a convenient term to refer to a group of babies whose deaths were neither witnessed nor explained by careful autopsies. There are probably hundreds of reasons that infants die unexpectedly, and we are never going to find a single cause to explain them all. No one knows exactly why

*Feldman, William and Mark E., *Lancet,* vol. 347 (April 20, 1996), p. 1057.

breastfeeding babies are less likely to be SIDS victims. It may merely be an association and not a case of cause and effect. However, if you are looking for another reason to breastfeed, this is one more to consider.

Advantages to your body. In the first few hours and days after your delivery, the sensation of your baby suckling at your breast will stimulate your uterus to contract vigorously. While this can be uncomfortable, it helps to expel the placenta, decreases the risk of excessive bleeding, and may help flatten your tummy a little more quickly.

Over the last fifteen years there have been numerous attempts to find a relationship between nursing and the risk of breast cancer. Unfortunately, as I am writing this chapter, there is not enough consistent data to allow us to claim that nursing provides significant protection against breast cancer.

Because breastfeeding drains nutrients, such as calcium, from your body and transfers them to your baby, some doctors have been concerned that nursing may actually contribute to osteoporosis. Fortunately, recent experiments have demonstrated that after weaning, your body will replenish its calcium supplies if you eat a nutritonally sound and adequate diet.

You may have heard that breastfeeding will provide you with a natural method of birth control. While it is true that nursing usually delays the reestablishment of your menstrual cycle, **do not count on breastfeeding for contraception.** It just isn't reliable. I have worked with scores of families who inadvertently found themselves with a toddler and an infant at the same time because they had relied exclusively on the "contraceptive" effect of nursing.

It's cheaper. With the cost of formula for a year estimated to be about $800 or $1000, you can see why breastfeeding may be less costly. Of course you will be eating and drinking more to maintain your milk supply, but I can't imagine that your expanded appetite will push your food bill up more than a few hundred dollars. Personally, I would much rather spend my money on something I can eat and enjoy, rather than have a large part of my income line the pockets of the formula manufacturers' CEOs.

You may realize some financial savings because nursing is often the "healthier" way to feed babies. For example, a large health maintenance organization estimated that formula-fed infants generated about $1,400 more in nonwell baby visit charges than children who were breastfed (another survey estimated about $400). One researcher estimated that if all infants in this country were entirely breastfed for their first twelve weeks, we would save more than $2 billion in the cost of illness alone.

Of course there are so many factors that contribute to your child's wellness that it would be foolish to count on saving a thousand dollars in medical expenses because you are nursing. However, you can be reasonably confident that breastfeeding probably won't be the more expensive way to feed your baby.

IF YOU HAVE A PREMATURE BABY, THE ADVANTAGES ARE EVEN GREATER

If your child is born prematurely, he is nutritionally disadvantaged. He no longer has your placenta to provide him with the critical nutrients that he needs to continue his growth and development. His immature gastrointestinal system may be injured by attempts to feed him before it is ready to safely digest foreign proteins. Premature babies are also more vulnerable to infection, and breastmilk may help reduce this risk.

I explained earlier that the data demonstrating the benefits of breastfeeding are not overwhelming for children who are born in societies of plenty. The advantages for premature infants, on the other hand, are more dramatic. Even if you are unsure if you want to continue nursing, these benefits may be so critical to the survival of your premature infant that I urge you pump your breasts while he is still in the intensive care nursery. This will allow you to feel like you are doing something (and you are) at a time when you may be feeling helpless. (See Appendix 3, "Nursing Your Premature Infant.")

4

I'm Afraid I Won't Like
Breastfeeding Because . . .

Although public health officials are eager to publicize the benefits of breastfeeding, not surprisingly, they seldom comment on its perceived disadvantages. This practice of ignoring the challenges of nursing is a strategic error. Their promotional efforts would be much more effective if breastfeeding proponents confronted the negative perceptions up front, because almost every rumored disadvantage of nursing I can think of has an obvious and practical solution. Unfortunately, these solutions are seldom discussed because breastfeeding advocates have preferred to pretend that breastfeeding simply has no downside.

I am sure that if you have watched other women nurse or listened to them discuss their breastfeeding experiences, you have already compiled a list of nursing cons all your own. Before we go any further let's take a look at them and see how many we can find simple solutions for.

Being my baby's only nutritional source makes me nervous. Though being completely responsible for every ounce your three-month-old baby has gained is an accomplishment you can be proud of, the realization that your child is wholly dependent upon your breast milk for his subsistence can be unsettling. Not every woman worries about being her baby's sole nutritional source, but I think most do. It is natural to worry and the responsibility is worth discussing.

You may have heard or read of frightening cases in which

babies who were being breastfed nearly starved to death because their mothers' milk supplies were inadequate. Yes, these cases have occurred, even in affluent suburbia, but they are extremely rare and, in every instance I am aware of, the situation could have been prevented by appropriately timed trips (not just phone calls) to a pediatrician's office.

If you follow the recommendations in *The Maternity Leave Breastfeeding Plan*, you won't have to worry about your baby not getting enough milk. At each step along the way I will encourage you to visit the pediatrician to have your baby weighed. I will continually remind you to not be embarrassed to visit the doctor frequently if you are worried. While phone calls can be a good way to gather information, they can sometimes provide false reassurance. Rely instead on your pediatrician's trained eyes and the scale in her office.

And remember there is always formula. We are no longer hunter-gatherers roaming the African plains foraging for food. Our babies don't have to starve when there is a drought or the berry crop is poor. Scientists have developed a reasonable substitute for breast milk so that if for some reason your body can't keep up with your baby's nutritional needs, you can zip down to the convenience store and buy a can of formula.

So please don't worry about being the sole nutritional source for your baby. Enjoy the sense of accomplishment as you watch your baby grow, and remember that the scale in your pediatrician's office and the cans of formula on the shelves in the grocery store will always be there if and when you need them.

I've heard that breastfeeding babies sleep less than those who are bottlefed. Yes, that is true. In the first month or two, breastfed babies on average will tend to feed a bit more often than their bottlefed counterparts. Breast milk is digested faster than formula. It is only natural that in the beginning your baby will probably want to feed more often. However, many, if not most, of the horror stories you have heard from and about women who have become exhausted and seriously sleep deprived while nursing are probably examples of situations in which mothers have allowed themselves to be used as pacifiers.

One of the cornerstones of *The Maternity Leave Breastfeeding Plan* is a commitment on my part to steer you clear of this trap. As early as the second or third week after delivery, we will begin laying the groundwork of a strategy that will allow your baby to learn to put himself to sleep. Once you are no longer a required element of his bedtime ritual, your baby will sleep longer, waking less often for non-nutritive "feedings" (unnecessary snacks), and you will be much less likely to feel ruled by your baby's sleeping and feeding schedules.

In more than twenty-five years of watching mothers breastfeed, it has become obvious that women who have avoided becoming pacifiers for their babies nurse longer, and, more important, are happier and more contented with their breastfeeding experiences. If your breastfeeding plan includes continuing to nurse when you return to work, you must avoid becoming a pacifier. There is no other way to make it succeed, unless you can work at home.

Parenting is going to rob you of sleep no matter how you slice it. However, breastfeeding won't compound the deficit, if you pay careful attention to managing your child's sleep from the beginning. *The Maternity Leave Breastfeeding Plan* will show you how to go about it.

I know I won't feel comfortable nursing in public. The sight of a woman breastfeeding her baby on a shopping mall bench is becoming more commonplace, but there are still many people in this country who feel that nursing should not be a public event. Some of these less enlightened critics would even go so far as to describe the practice as "tasteless" or "disgusting."

Our society has come a long way in its acceptance of the unclothed body, but, like it or not, the human breast is still considered to be primarily a sexual object. Although in some parts of the world women are seen bare breasted in public, you and I live in North America, and our puritanical history is not going to disappear overnight.

If the thought of nursing your baby in public doesn't bother you, then you need only deal with the occasional rude comment from the less-liberated passerby. However, I suspect that you won't feel completely comfortable breastfeeding in the presence of strangers or even around some of the members of your own family. Don't worry. That kind of shyness is perfectly appropriate in our society and should not interfere with a chance of having a positive nursing experience, because *you don't have to breastfeed in public.*

Why not? Again, the answer has to do with sleep and its relationship to breastfeeding. In the first three months of life your child may be nursing every two or three hours, and he should be sleeping the rest of the time, between fourteen and sixteen hours a day. Almost all of this sleeping should be done in his crib because most children sleep poorly in strange places, and consequently they may become overtired, overstimulated, and irritable if they spend too much time away from home. Furthermore, with crowds come germs, and breastfed or not, infants are still very vulnerable to infection.

In other words, for the first three months there is really very little reason for your child to be breastfed in public because he should be home sleeping most of the time. His infrequent trips out of the house will be to the pediatrician's office for checkups and the occasional visit to Grandma's house. While this may sound like a rather conservative recommendation, I have found that sticking close to home, away from the germ-infested and chaotic outside world, for the first three months will help your child to remain healthy and contented.

As he gets older, your baby will become more social. He will be feeding much less often and won't be sleeping quite so much. He will be ready for short trips out of the house. However, you should still keep his sleep needs high on the priority list. Public appearances should be scheduled around naps. If you are uncomfortable nursing in public, appearances can be worked around his feedings. If you introduce a bottle when he is a month old, he may be willing to take one as an alternative. If you are careful to avoid the pacifier trap, you will have many fewer nursings to work around because your baby will be nursing only when he is hungry, not when he is tired.

The bottom line is that if you don't want to breastfeed in public, you won't have to. In fact, if you have put your child's health and sleep needs appropriately high on your priority list, there will be very few occasions when nursing in front of strangers will be necessary.

It won't fit into my work schedule. Yes, there is a good chance that once you return to work, you won't have the time or the energy to continue to breastfeed. However, there are enough good reasons to nurse your baby for his first three months that the likelihood that you will have to wean him when you return to your job should not deter you from starting. In fact, that is one of the reasons that I decided to write *The Maternity Leave Breastfeeding Plan.* By the time you have finished reading the first few chapters, I am confident that you will realize that nursing your baby for his first ninety days is not only a worthwhile but also a very achievable goal. You may also discover that by careful attention to managing your baby's sleep schedules, you may actually be able to continue to breastfeed when you return to work.

Weaning will be difficult and painful. I suspect you already know that if you decide to limit your nursing to your baby's first ninety days, you will probably be ending his breastfeeding experience before he would otherwise choose to stop. In other words *you* are the one who will have to initiate the weaning process.

There are infants who inexplicably decide to stop nursing on their own at two or three months of age, but most would prefer to continue until they are at least six or seven months old and they have developed an affinity for solid foods. Of course there are a few children who enjoy breastfeeding so much that they want to keep at it well beyond their second birthday.

I won't lie to you. When you wean your baby before he wants to stop, regardless of whether it is simply because you aren't enjoying nursing any longer or because circumstances give you no choice, it is going to be a sad day (or days) for both you and your baby. However, if done properly and without vacillation, the process will go much more quickly and easily than you may have been led to believe.

If you have been careful to avoid becoming your baby's pacifier, weaning will be much easier. Although it may not be very comforting to your ego, your baby will quickly accept bottles of formula if you aren't available to feed him. Even the most stubborn baby will take only a day or two to read the handwriting on the wall, if his primary purpose for nursing is nutritional. However, if his mother's breast has become an integral part of his going-to-sleep ritual, weaning is going to be a longer and more difficult process.

Arriving at the decision to stop nursing can be very difficult, and the process of weaning itself is seldom easy, but by following *The Maternity Leave Breastfeeding Plan* you will find that it is manageable and hopefully easier than you might fear it to be. If you wish, you can leap ahead to chapters 21 and 22 for a preview of what you can expect. I hope you will realize that though you may have to stop nursing your baby before he wants to quit, that's no reason to avoid breastfeeding altogether.

I've heard horror stories about sore nipples and leaking breasts. Yes, many women experience nipple soreness in the first few days after delivery. The discomfort is usually temporary and can sometimes be prevented by careful attention to proper nursing technique. Though rare, a few women, many of whom have preexisting skin conditions, have persistent nipple soreness.

The bottom line is that while no one can promise you that your breastfeeding experience will be painfree, there are strategies for minimizing your discomfort. These have been woven into chapters 9 and 12, and I am confident that when you look back on your three-month nursing experience, you won't think of it as ninety days of physical torture.

Most women experience periods when their breasts produce more milk than their baby can drink and some of the excess drips from their nipples. This mismatch between supply and demand usually occurs in the first few weeks and resolves quickly as a mother's body adapts to a baby's needs. Many women will leak milk when they hear their baby cry or even when they hear any baby cry. Some mothers need only think about their baby to initiate their let-down reflex. While it can be embarrassing, uncontrolled milk releases become less frequent as the weeks go by, and I can't recall any mother who has chosen to stop nursing because her breasts were leaking excessively.

This short discussion may not include all your worries about breastfeeding. However, I suspect that as you continue to read *The Maternity Leave Breastfeeding Plan* you will encounter sections that address most, if not all of your concerns. The more you learn, the less you will have to worry about.

5

AN ENERGY CRISIS IN THE MAKING

While breast milk may be the best first food you can offer your child, it is expensive. I'm not talking about dollars and cents. In fact, you can expect to save money in the first three months that you nurse your baby. The cost I am referring to is in energy expenditure.

Considering that most of the lactating mothers I know complain that they feel tired most of the time, I have always suspected that breastfeeding was a drain on a woman's energy reserves. However, it wasn't until I read *A Natural History of Parenting* (Three Rivers Press, 1998) by naturalist Susan Allport that I realized just how critical the energy cost of lactation is to the survival of all mammalian species, including our own.

Ms. Allport observes that mammary glands (breasts) are far less efficient at supplying nutrients than is the placenta. She notes that some scientists even view the mammary gland as a parasite on the mammalian female because nursing's energy cost is so high. While this may not be the most appealing image, the point is that nursing comes at a price your body must pay.

The higher energy cost of lactation means that while you may have been able to work right up until the day you delivered, you may not have the stamina to continue nursing when you return to your job. Regardless of how motivated you are, biology has dealt you a difficult hand to play.

Are there solutions to this inevitable energy crisis? Yes! One strategy that other mammalian species have employed is to assign helpers to assist the lactating female in finding food and conserving energy. In some cases this may be another female or group of females who can help her care for her offspring. In other species this helper is the male who fathered the baby. He may hunt or forage for food and protect the mother and infant from predators and other environmental threats.

There are obvious parallels between these strategies and your situation. During the first few weeks after you deliver, you will probably be lavished with offers of help from your husband, mother, mother-in-law, sister, and friends. Everyone expects you to be exhausted during the immediate postpartum period. However, in short order they will expect you to resume many, if not all, of your old responsibilities. After all, you aren't pregnant anymore. But what everyone has overlooked is that you are still nursing, and as you and I now understand, this means that the energy demands on your body are even greater than when you were pregnant.

The bottom line is that if you are hoping to continue nursing when your maternity leave is over, you must reach out to some of those helping hands who flocked to your assistance immediately after you delivered. I hope that your husband is planning to assume some nontraditional roles, such as shopping and cleaning the house, because he is the obvious first choice as an energy-saving assistant. You and he can read in chapters 9 and 10 some specific suggestions on how a team effort can improve your chances of being able to nurse adequately after you return to work.

Unfortunately most women are not very successful in finding surrogates to assume their home-based responsibilities. A study published in 1998 found that working mothers spend thirty-two hours each week doing household chores and twenty-eight hours each week caring for children . . . a total of only seven hours per week less than women who were full-time stay-at-home mothers.

Don't allow yourself to fall into the if-she-can-do-it-I-can-do-it trap. Although lactation is a significant drain on every nursing mother's body, there are a few women who have been blessed with an unusual amount of stamina. These "super mothers" seem to be able to work full-time, chair the United Fund Drive, take continuing-education classes in Portuguese, and continue to nurse their babies. Women like this are made of a little different stuff than the rest of us and should be considered the Olympic athletes of the breastfeeding world.

Don't let an encounter with one of these Olympians dash your hopes of continuing to nurse when you return to work. It may not be as easy as you anticipated, but if it doesn't work out, you needn't feel that you are any less of a woman.

6

CAUGHT BETWEEN CYCLES, UNDERSTANDING YOUR PLACE IN HISTORY

As you prepare yourself for the challenge of breastfeeding in a society that can't honestly be described as "nursing-friendly," it may be of some small comfort to consider where you fit into the ebb and flow of the history of breastfeeding. While I am troubled by our society's eagerness to cast us as victims when our paths lead us into unfortunate circumstances, we do live our lives within the limits of our particular culture. We are not victims of our society, but products of the forces that it exerts upon us. This reality is certainly true of breastfeeding and its compatibility or incompatibility with work outside the home. If you were living in England in the seventeenth century, your attempts at combining nursing and employment would have been influenced by a different set of factors. Some would have been positive, some negative, some very similar to those that will shape your breastfeeding career today.

Before I began doing my research for this book, I assumed that we were living at the bottom of a long and steady decline in the popularity of breastfeeding that began in prehistoric times, when all of our ancestors were forced to nurse their children or face extinction. Nothing could be further from the truth. For at least the last thousand years women and the societies that they live in have run hot and cold on the notion of breastfeeding. In mid-eighteenth-century Paris breastfeeding had become so unfashionable that 50 percent of the infants were sent to the countryside to be raised by wet nurses. This decline in popularity became so profound that by 1780 only about 10 percent of babies born in Paris were nursed in their own homes. However, the end of the century saw a dramatic change in philosophy and political attitude toward breastfeeding. By 1801 half of all Parisian babies were again being nursed by their mothers.

During the Italian Renaissance, artists depicted the Madonna nursing the infant Jesus. Some art historians have proposed that these paintings represented an effort by the Church to encourage upper-class Florentine women to begin to nurse their babies and stop the practice of sending their children to the country for their first two years.

Why would French and Italian women need to be reminded that nursing their own children was better than literally "farming them out"? Male-dominated societies have at times sought to preserve a woman's breasts for the enjoyment of her husband. For some upper-class women breastfeeding was seen as an unnecessary interruption in their sexual and social lives. Nursing can be time consuming, painful, and confining, and it will temporarily alter the appearance of a woman's breasts. It is not surprising that many women would willingly yield to the societal forces that discouraged the practice. We certainly saw this trend repeat itself in North America when infant formulas became practical and readily available in the early twentieth century.

During the sixteenth and seventeenth centuries Dutch medical, religious, and moral authorities consistently supported breastfeeding. Paintings from that period make it very clear that a woman's place was in the home and that one of her primary obligations was to nurse her baby. It is tempting to allow these beautiful pictures of domestic tranquillity to lull us into believing that this was the golden age of breastfeeding. Remember that these women were more or less confined to the home. However, it probably was comforting for a nursing mother to be surrounded by a family and a society that was in agreement in its support of her breastfeeding.

You and I are living in North America at the turn of the twenty-first century, and we obviously don't have our act together when it comes to breastfeeding. On one hand those of us in the scientific community are telling women that breast milk is the best first food for their babies. On the other hand politicians have done very little to create any legal framework to support these same women's efforts at nursing. Our maternity leave policies are in the very early stages of development; most women can't negotiate an absence long enough to nurse their babies until they are ready for solid food. Our schizophrenic society monetarily rewards women for working away from home at the same time as it gives lip service to their attempts at continuing to breastfeed. The truth, of course, is that these two endeavors are often incompatible.

But here we are trapped in a society that at least for the moment is more than willing to make you feel guilty if you deprive your baby of your breast milk, but erects barriers for women who want to return to work and continue to nurse. You can whine about it and consider you and your baby victims of a society whose priorities are in disarray, or you can acknowledge the challenges and try to overcome them. The second path makes the most sense to me, and it is that approach that you will find as you read on.

If our society's schizophrenic approach to breastfeeding wasn't a big enough challenge, evolution has failed to keep pace with societal change. Biologists who study mammalian milk separate mammals into two distinct categories based on the nutritional composition of their milk. Human milk falls into the category in which the infants can nurse more or less continuously. The milk from continuous-feeding mammalian mothers is lower in fat and protein, and their offspring don't consume a large volume of milk in a single feeding. The other category includes mammals who nurse their offspring in bursts widely spaced throughout the day. This pattern is called spaced feeding.

When our species was evolving, mothers carried their infants with them as they scoured the countryside for food. The babies of nomadic hunter-gatherers were better off being continuous feeders, and the milk production of the mothers adapted to that situation. Obviously, that's not how we live today. The image of a woman driving a sport utility vehicle with her infant suckling at her breast just doesn't compute. While we may have begun as continuous feeders tens of thousands of years ago, we are now clearly spaced feeders even though the content of human milk is more appropriate to a continuous schedule.

Fortunately, most of our children have adapted easily to this mismatch between the kind of milk they are being fed and the schedule on which it is provided. However, it is likely that the colicky behavior and excessive spitting up that plagues some infants during their first three months is a consequence of being fed relatively large volumes of breast milk a few times a day. If they were allowed to take smaller feedings whenever they wished, these babies might not have what appear to be belly aches.

This disparity between the composition of human milk and the way in which we feed our babies seems to be of little consequence biologically. I mention it as just another example of how it is a mistake to assume that just because breastfeeding is the "natural" way to feed babies that it will mesh with our twenty-first-century North American lifestyle. We have come too far in too short a time to make it an easy fit.

7

How Long Should I Breastfeed My Baby?

Just like the decision to breastfeed, deciding when to stop is up to you entirely. You shouldn't feel pressured or coerced into nursing any longer than you want. There will be good days and bad days. When you feel that the negatives are outnumbering the positives, it is probably time to stop. However, I hope that by following the Maternity Leave Breastfeeding Plan you will avoid many of the pitfalls that made nursing so unpleasant for others that they couldn't wait to stop. For example, if we can keep you from becoming your baby's pacifier, you will be much less likely to feel fatigued or tied down, two of the most common complaints of breastfeeding mothers.

Even if nursing comes easily and you are skillful enough to avoid becoming a pacifier, you may not enjoy breastfeeding. It just may not be your cup of tea. Some women like the physical sensation of their baby suckling or feel empowered by being their child's sole nutritional source. Maybe you don't. That doesn't mean that there is anything wrong with you, but if you don't enjoy nursing, it is unlikely that you plan on breastfeeding until your child is eighteen months old. That's okay.

There are many factors to consider when you are deciding how long to nurse your baby. You have control over some, but not all of them. Before we consider some of these issues, remember that how you feed your baby is one of many parental responsibilities. I want you to breastfeed only as long as you feel it is a positive experience, and I don't want you to feel guilty when you finally wean your baby. You may feel sad that one chapter in your relationship with your baby has ended, but I don't want you to feel that you must continue to nurse just because someone else thinks you should.

Let's hear what the doctors say. In 1997 the American Academy of Pediatrics released a policy statement titled "Breastfeeding and the Use of Human Milk," which included two recommendations.* One was that "exclusive breastfeeding is ideal nutrition" for the first six months, and the other suggestion was that "breastfeeding continue for at least twelve months." Although this five-page statement offered numerous strategies to promote breastfeeding, this latter recommendation received most of the media attention. Our local newspaper headlined the Associated Press story MOTHERS URGED TO BREAST-FEED A YEAR (*Portland Press Herald,* December 3,1997).

While I am sure the committee that drafted the policy statement felt its document would encourage more women to breastfeed, the publicity surrounding its release may have had the opposite effect. You may find the notion of breastfeeding for at least twelve months so unappealing and unrealistic that you wonder if it is even worth starting. You may already know that your workplace and schedule are not breastfeeding-friendly, and perhaps can't imagine how you could ever continue nursing when your three-month maternity leave has ended. The American Academy of Pediatrics didn't intend to send you on a guilt trip, but their guidelines may have unwittingly done just that.

Let's look at some other medical sources for more realistic guidelines. Unfortunately it is hard to get a straight answer because many of the studies have yielded conflicting results. Others have been criticized for "flawed methodologies." Regarding SIDS and allergy prevention, the data is so murky that it's of no use at all to us.

---

* The American Academy of Pediatrics, "Breastfeeding and the Use of Human Milk," *Pediatrics,* vol. 100 (6) (December 1997), pp. 1034-1039.

However, when it comes to protection against infection we may find a somewhat clearer answer. In 1997, scientists working for the CDC (Centers for Disease Control) and the FDA (Federal Drug Administration) conducted a survey of more than three thousand households and concluded sensibly that "The more breast milk an infant receives in the first six months, the less likely that he or she will develop diarrhea or ear infection."* They also observed that, "in a society where the mother has to meet many responsibilities in addition to feeding her infant, exclusive breastfeeding may not always be practical. . . . [B]reastfeeding is not an all-or-none phenomenon; the more breast milk an infant receives in the first six months of life the better."

However, a survey of asthmatic women performed in Arizona revealed that the longer they breastfed their baby the more likely their child would develop asthma. Nine percent of children who never breastfed developed asthma; among children who nursed for longer than four months the asthma rate was nearly six times greater. No one can explain these unexpected results, but it does point out that more breast milk may not always be better. You must look at your own unique situation; when the negatives outweigh the positives it is time to stop.

In other words, do the best you can. If you can breastfeed your baby exclusively for the first three months, that's wonderful. If you have to supplement with formula, don't feel guilty. Even if you have nursed your baby for only a month, you have provided him with an excellent start on life. Although the research data to support this position is scanty, I think it is safe to say that the first few months of nursing are the most important. Keep in mind this is not a contest. No pediatrician I know is handing out stripes to wear on your sleeve for each month you breastfeed your baby.

Should I try to continue breastfeeding after I return to work? I have already given you the statistics. The odds are stacked against

*Paula Scariati et al. "A Longitudinal Analysis of Infant Morbidity and the Extent of Breastfeeding in the United States." *Pediatrics,* vol. 99 (6) (June 1997), p. e5.

you, but if it is something you want to try, I will be giving you tips on strategy and words of encouragement when things aren't going well. The bottom line still remains the same. When the negatives outweigh the positives it's time to stop. If despite our best laid plans, you find that the combination of work and nursing is leaving you a zombie at the end of the day, then it is probably time to wean your baby.

Some jobs are so inherently incompatible with nursing that you may already know that you will be weaning your child when you return to work. For example, if you are a flight attendant on the San Francisco to New York run, pumping and storing breast milk is going to be very difficult. On the other hand your job may allow you the opportunity to continue breastfeeding, but you may be concerned about the energy drain. Before you make the decision, read and reread Chapter 8, "Preparing Your Mind and Adopting an Attitude," and "Creating a Nursing-Friendly Workplace" (page 62). Learn as much as you can about breastfeeding. Make a *realistic* assessment of your job, your strengths, and vulnerabilities. Set some reasonable goals and then establish a plan for reaching them. By the time you have finished Chapter 9, you should have a pretty good idea where you are going.

Your baby and your body may not cooperate. After reading *The Maternity Leave Breastfeeding Plan* and talking to several friends and co-workers who have breastfed, you may decide that you are going to nurse your baby for at least six months. This will probably require that you pump and store breast milk when you return to work after your maternity leave has ended. You suspect it will be a hassle, but you have decided to go for it anyway.

Your nursing partner may not see it the same way you do. When offered an increasing number of bottle feedings, some babies will begin to balk at the breast. Sometimes the baby is impatient and prefers the faster flow of a bottle nipple. In your case it may be that your baby is upset by what he perceives to be instability. It is as though he is saying, "Hey, Mom, which is it going to be? You or the bottle? I won't do both." Fortunately, most babies enjoy breastfeeding so much that they are willing to put up with switching back and forth. However, I am warning you not to count on it.

A more likely scenario is that your body decides it just can't make milk and go back to work at the same time. It's not that your mind isn't committed to the plan. You may be steadfastly committed to continuing nursing when you return to work, but after your body recalculates its energy supplies, it realizes that to keep going it will have to cut back somewhere. Unfortunately, it decides to protect you and decrease, or even stop, milk production.

Sometimes this decrease in milk production occurs because your body doesn't respond well to the artificial suction of a breast pump. It may interpret the decrease in true nursings as a decrease in demand, and therefore produce less milk. There isn't much you can do about this. You can try a different pump or pumping more often. You can hold a picture of your baby on your lap while you are pumping, though these strategies are limited in their effectiveness.

More often, the decrease in milk supply is a direct result of the fatigue that occurs when every woman goes back to work. You may have to accept this as a sad reality of life in the twenty-first century. However, I hope that after reading *The Maternity Leave Breastfeeding Plan* you will understand how important sleep management is for successful parenting and will have learned some strategies for keeping you and your baby well rested. I can't promise you that your body can keep making enough milk when you return to work, but you can give it your best shot by avoiding serious sleep deprivation.

Will it be hard to stop nursing? Yes, it could be, but it won't be the most difficult transition you will ever have to make. You may find that despite your apprehensions and preconceptions you really enjoy breastfeeding. Although you plan to nurse only until you return to work or until your baby turns six months, you may discover that breastfeeding hasn't been that difficult and that you look forward to those opportunities for closeness.

If you want to continue nursing until your child is two or three years old, that's fine. However, when you no longer find it pleasurable, it is time to stop. I don't want you to keep breastfeeding because you are afraid to stop or are unsure exactly how to go about it. To help you through the process I have devoted an entire section of Chapter 21 to weaning. Together we will explore the emotions that can complicate this transition and some strategies that can smooth your path.

A popular and realistic scenario. I have warned you that the unpredictability of biologic processes such as breastfeeding make it dangerous to set firm timetables and goals for your breastfeeding career. However, you may feel more comfortable if you have a rough road map in hand as you begin this journey into the unknown. Your path will be dictated by the circumstances of your life, but here is a scenario that has been popular with the mothers in my practice:

- First month. Committed to getting a good start and introducing your baby to the concept of sleep independence. Offer a rare relief bottle to prevent maternal fatigue.

- At one month. Begin to introduce a bottle on a regular basis. This could be as often as once a day, or as infrequently as once a week. However, there is no guarantee your baby will accept the bottle the first few attempts (see Chapter 20).

- At two months. If you are thinking about returning to work, begin to pump and save milk (optional).

- At three months. Return to work if you must. This will probably mean either pumping or giving your baby formula. He *will* take a bottle at this point, even though he may have rejected it before. Hunger and thirst are powerful motivators (see Chapter 20).

- At four months. Begin to offer solid food (see Chapter 22).

- <u>At five months.</u> Introduce a cup (see Chapter 22).

- <u>At eight or nine months.</u> If your child has been skillful at learning to drink from a cup and enjoys solid food *and* you have avoided becoming his pacifier, he may have begun to wean himself already. At least all the groundwork has been laid for you to initiate weaning and have it completed by the time he is a year old, or earlier if you wish.

8

Preparing Your Mind and Adopting an Attitude

If you want your nursing experience to be a positive one, it helps to begin with an attitude that will not only help you endure the challenges but also those inevitable, unpredictable wrinkles that will occur along the way. I could simply admonish you to cleanse your mind of negative thoughts and adopt a "can-do" attitude. However, you know as well as I, getting into the correct frame of mind is never as easy as repeating the mantra "I think I can, I think I can, I think I can." Neither the human mind nor the biologic process of breastfeeding is that simple.

Like every other woman, you will arrive at parenthood with your own unique collection of strengths, weaknesses, fears, and assumptions. While I can predict that motherhood is going to be exhausting, I cannot predict how you will respond when the challenge begins. And, for that matter, neither can you. Harriet Lerner, psychologist and author of *The Mother Dance: How Children Change Your Life* (HarperCollins, 1998), has said, "The thing about motherhood is that we don't have a clue what it will evoke in us until it is our turn." Another psychologist, Brenda Hunter, has referred to the event as a "psychic earthquake."

Although there is no single "correct" frame of mind, there are several attitude issues to consider. Drawing on the work of psychologists and nurse-educators as well as my own experiences with thousands of breastfeeding mothers over the last thirty years, I can offer you some suggestions of how, by adopting a more nursing-friendly philosophy, you can improve your chances of success.

I'm not going to try to change who you are. If you are timid, I'm not going to ask you to become a risk-taking daredevil. If you are an intense type A person, I am not going to suggest that you sit back and passively let the world pummel you. However, I hope that after reading this chapter you can tweak your approach to life here and there to make breastfeeding not only work, but work so well that you will want to do it again.

Accept the uncertainty of nursing. Breastfeeding, like all biologic processes, comes with no guarantees. You can do everything by the book and still end up supplementing with formula. Large breasts don't guarantee success, nor do small breasts necessarily produce less milk. There is no way of knowing whether you will be able to provide your baby with enough milk to thrive. Not every woman can become pregnant and not every mother can breastfeed. No one can tell if you're going to be plagued by breast infections or if your breasts will leak excessively. Although you roll the dice and take your chances, the good news is that the odds are heavily in your favor.

As researcher Dr. Jane Bottorff has written, "Every mother knows that choosing to breastfeed is a journey into the unknown." We all have trouble taking those first tentative steps on an unfamiliar path, but if you happen to be a "control freak" like me, it is even more difficult to trust your fate and that of your baby to a process with no guarantee of success.

Before you decide to take this leap of faith, let's take a step back and look at what, if any, real risks you will be taking. There really aren't any. Remember, you live in twenty-first-century North America. There is a grocery store within a few miles of your home stocked with breastmilk substitutes that have been fed to millions of infants. You have a doctor to call if you are concerned that your baby isn't getting enough milk, and you have phone and transportation to get to the doctor's office. What is there to worry about?

You may have read frightening newspaper accounts of babies who have starved because they weren't getting enough breastmilk.

On closer examination you will discover that these were all tragedies that could have easily been avoided if the family had been able to maintain a close relationship with a physician and visited the office instead of merely relying on telephone advice. If you follow the suggestions in this book, namely calling your doctor and scheduling frequent office visits so that your baby can be weighed and examined (see Chapter 16), you won't have to worry that your baby will suffer from an inadequate milk supply. If the pediatrician you have selected is unwilling to see your child, promptly seek a second or third opinion.

There is no way to remove the uncertainty that is inherent in breastfeeding. It might be easier if your breasts were transparent so that you could watch the milk level go down during feedings. This might provide you with some of the visual reassurance that mothers who bottlefeed can enjoy, but obviously it isn't going to happen. Accept the uncertainty of breastfeeding, but remember there are scores of us standing by, ready to help.

Don't blame breastfeeding for changes in your life that are primarily the consequence of motherhood. You may have heard some mothers complain that they felt tied down while they were nursing. Other women are uncomfortable with the thought that only they can feed their babies. The feeling of total responsibility can be lonely and frightening.

However, these are emotions that bottlefeeding mothers feel as well. In describing what it feels like to become a mother, Harriet Lerner has said, "You discover you are open to a wider range of emotions." She adds, "You wrap feelings of guilt and inadequacy around you like a familiar blanket, even if they are feelings you never had before."

Of course breastfeeding can intensify these emotions because you don't have a bottle of formula to act as a thin layer of insulation from the cold reality of parenting. However, don't think that by bottlefeeding you will avoid the feelings of responsibility that are part and parcel of motherhood. With that first cry in the delivery room your life has changed forever. There is no going back.

The reality may sink in a little more quickly if you breastfeed, but no matter how you feed your baby, there's no escaping the responsibility you've taken on. You are caring for another person's life.

Learn when to trust Mother Nature. While breastfeeding is the natural way to feed your baby, that doesn't mean that it always works. For the most part you can rely on your own instincts and those of your baby to guide you in the right direction. This is particularly true in the first few days when you are wondering how often to feed your baby. If he is crying, he is probably hungry.

However, there are other situations when you may not be able to completely trust Mother Nature's guidance. "Attachment" is just the beginning. Although we might like to assume that you and your baby will "naturally" figure out how to get his mouth attached to your breast in such a way that will guarantee optimal milk transfer, sometimes it doesn't happen. Putting your nipple into your baby's mouth is not always a hand-in-glove process. You may need to ask a nurse or lactation consultant for help.

In other words you can trust Mother Nature to make breastfeeding work, but not blindly. The fact that millions of women around the world are nursing successfully every day should comfort and encourage you as you face the scariest parts of breastfeeding, such as waiting for your milk to come in. However, continue to ask your support group for reassurance and advice. Even Mother Nature needs some help from time to time.

Set realistic goals with several alternative plans. You may have already decided that you want to continue nursing after you return to work. That's great, but wait until you have finished reading this book before you decide to firmly establish this as a goal. When you learn what it requires in terms of energy and effort to create a breastfeeding-friendly work environment, you may realize that there is little chance for success, or that it comes at a cost you are unwilling to pay. This will mean looking at yourself honestly. Ask yourself, "Am I a person who tires easily?" "Will I have the stamina to nurse and go to work?" "Can I be assertive enough to go into my boss's office and ask for a comfortable place to nurse?"

Don't let me discourage you from setting goals that currently seem just a bit out of reach. As long as you can accept that breastfeeding comes with no guarantees, *and* you have some alternative plans in mind, you will do just fine. For example, you may be lucky enough to have a daycare center so close to work that you can zip over and nurse your baby several times a day. Then again that center may close a few weeks after your baby starts to get comfortable with the staff. It happens. Now, you must either find daycare that is close by or start pumping at work, which was certainly not part of Plan A. If you have alternate plans in place for when something like this happens, you will be well on the way to salvaging your breastfeeding career.

As you make arrangements to support your long-term plan, ask yourself "what if" questions at each step along the way: "What if I can't pump enough milk?" "What if we get so busy in the office that I can't work just part-time for the next six months?" You don't need to have a firm Plan B in place for every situation. Just having thought about an alternative is sufficient to keep you from being derailed by an unexpected stone on the tracks.

Avoid specific goals such as "I am going to nurse my baby for nine months." There are so many variables that can affect the process that you run a substantial risk of disappointment. Your primary goal should be the simplest and most realistic. "I'm going to continue to breastfeed my baby as long as both of us want to do it." Then you can begin to implement strategies to make that happen regardless of the expected and unexpected difficulties ahead.

Don't think too much about "trying" to breastfeed. Just do it! It may just be another round in the semantics game, but you will be much more likely to have a rewarding nursing experience if you avoid saying, "I am going to *try* to breastfeed." Instead, simply announce, "I am going to nurse my baby." While "trying" does acknowledge the uncertainty that is inherent in breastfeeding, it sends a negative message to everyone, including yourself. Don't hesitate to share your apprehensions with anyone who will listen. Hopefully, they can offer you some helpful advice, support, and reassurance. But start off with the commitment that you are going to do it. You don't know how long you are going to breastfeed, but right now you are assembling all of the resources you will need to make it work.

Avoid the "F-word." For many breastfeeding advocates the F-word to avoid is *formula* (see Chapter 15). However, the one that I want us both to avoid is *failure.* While I used the word in "Do We Really Need Another Book About Breastfeeding?" you won't read it again. On the other hand, I won't hesitate to use the word *success,* and I will refer to *positive nursing experiences* from time to time. Again, it may be just semantics, but I have written this book to be mother-friendly, and referring to you as a failure just doesn't fit.

Let's keep our conversation, and the conversations you have with yourself, moving in a positive direction. You are going to (not just try to) breastfeed. It may not work out, but not because there is something wrong with you. You didn't fail. You just stopped nursing. You will still be a mother and a damn good one at that.

Don't necessarily play by the rules. Because there aren't any. Breastfeeding can work even if you follow none of the suggestions in this book. There are no absolutes and no rules. For example, even though I will warn you to avoid offering your newborn a pacifier until he is several weeks old, I know hundreds of babies who were given pacifiers on their first day of life who still became excellent nursers.

Women often fear that they will have to severely restrict their diet while they are nursing. That's just not true. You will probably be able to eat anything you want and still have an occasional alcoholic beverage while you are breastfeeding. There are only a handful of standard medications that might get into your breast milk and harm your baby (see Appendix 2). Similarly, there are very few medical conditions and treatments that are not compatible with nursing.

Please don't accept my advice or that of any other breastfeeding advocate as gospel. Create your own unique experience by combining what you have read with your own common sense. Relax. Don't invest precious energy worrying about whether you are doing it the "wrong" way. There is not one correct way to breastfeed. It's whatever works for you and your baby.

Don't confuse intensity with positivity. You may have already decided to breastfeed and you may plan to commit all of your energy into making it work. I am pleased with your decision, but I am a little worried about the intensity of your commitment. Nursing is one of those activities, like dancing or sex, that the harder you try, the more difficult they are to master. Your tension will be transmitted to your partner, your baby in this case, and can interfere with his attempts to make the process work. The stress of trying too hard can also interfere with your ability to let down milk.

I know that telling you to relax is like telling you to be spontaneous, now! It just doesn't work that way. Struggle to maintain your positivity without being too intense. As expert Sheila Kitzinger has observed, "determination cannot itself produce milk and is in fact not a good basis for the relaxed and casual feeling which is dominant . . . where breastfeeding is most successful."

Remember, millions of women each year successfully breastfeed their babies. You will be surrounded by people who will support your efforts, and I will help you string a safety net beneath you and your baby, should things not work out.

Preparing your body. Preparing your mind for breastfeeding is far more important than preparing your body. However, there are some things you can do to ready yourself physiologically for lactation. You have heard much about them before. Eat a healthy diet. Get plenty of sleep and fresh air. Exercise in moderation. These practices will ensure that your body stays healthy during your pregnancy, and they will prepare you for the added physical demands of breastfeeding.

The getting-plenty-of-sleep part is the one you are probably having the most trouble with. Most pregnant women don't sleep well as they approach their delivery date. It just happens. However, do whatever you can to keep your days as restful as possible. Interrupted sleep won't allow you to replace the energy drained off by a hectic day. Move fatigue prevention nearer to the top of your priority list. Staying well rested is important and will be critical once you are a nursing mother.

Preparing your nipples for breastfeeding must be done carefully. The obstetricians I know feel that prenatal nipple preparation is seldom effective in preventing sore nipples. In fact, many of them are concerned that excessive nipple stimulation by handling or toweling could trigger uterine contractions that might result in premature labor. Most nipple soreness seems to be related to factors that occur after the baby is born. The positioning of your baby's mouth and the care of your nipples once you have started nursing (Chapters 11 and 12) are probably much more important than prenatal preparation.

Ask your obstetrician or a lactation consultant to check to see if you have excessively flat or inverted nipples. They may suggest that you wear a special cup in your bra to encourage your nipples to stand out. However, this should be done very carefully and stopped promptly if you are experiencing more than the usual number of uterine contractions. Nipple rolling and manipulation should definitely be avoided.

For most women nipple preparation should simply consist of spending part of each day braless. The gentle friction of a T-shirt against your nipples as you move about will help toughen your nipples but won't stimulate them enough to trigger uterine contractions.

9

A Plan for the Three Months *Before* You Deliver

I probably should have titled this book *The Six Month Breastfeeding Plan,* because although most of the women reading it will be nursing for the three months of their maternity leave, preparations for a successful breastfeeding experience should really begin about three months *before* delivery. The ebb and flow of hormones associated with pregnancy will take care of preparing your breasts for milk production. However, there are several important tasks that you should be working on before D-day. You should be assembling your support group to help you during the first two critical weeks. You should also be looking for daycare that will fit into your breastfeeding plans. If you are thinking about continuing to nurse when you go back to work, you should be negotiating schedules and looking for a space that can serve as a comfortable and private place to pump. Finally, you should be settling into a frame of mind that will allow you to accept breastfeeding's unpredictability and surmount its challenges. If you wait until after you deliver, you will have neither the time nor the energy to complete these tasks. *The Maternity Leave Breastfeeding Plan* can help you have a very enjoyable and rewarding nursing experience, but you must plan ahead if it is going to work.

GATHERING YOUR SUPPORT GROUP

While some women are lucky enough to master breastfeeding on their own, most new mothers need help to get the process going smoothly. Even gorillas who are nursing their babies for the first time often require the assistance of an older and more experienced female to succeed. Just because breastfeeding is the more "natural" way to feed your baby doesn't mean it happens by itself. You will probably need help, and now is the time to begin assembling your support group. Don't wait until after your delivery to start. By the time you find it, it may be too late.

In some societies new mothers are customarily provided with a doula, a woman who provides support and education after delivery. While some hospitals and birthing centers are beginning to offer "doula services," the practice is not widespread, and you will probably need to create your own support network by drawing on several different sources. This will take time, and you may need to interview several people before you decide who to include on your list of helpers.

QUALITIES TO CONSIDER

Knowledgeable. There are many different ways to breastfeed successfully. It is important to find someone who knows enough about nursing to help you avoid the common pitfalls. Although he may be your best friend, don't count on your husband as a *knowledgeable* supporter. If you were breastfed, your mother could be a good source of information. Lactation consultants and obstetrical and pediatric nurses are the best sources of breastfeeding facts.

Supportive. When the going gets tough you'll want to be surrounded by people who believe that breastfeeding is important and want to do whatever they can to help you and your baby. I hope that your husband fits this description. Sadly, some men view their wife's breasts as their own property and see the baby as competition. Others aren't convinced that breastfeeding is the best way to feed babies, particularly when they see how thin and watery breast milk looks. Ask your spouse to read this book along with you, so that you are both literally "on the same page" when it comes to the value of breastfeeding and the strategies that are necessary to make it work.

Your best female friend (e.g., your sister or your best friend) and your mother may also be your biggest supporters. On the other hand, if your mother thinks that breastfeeding is "just one of those yuppie fads," it would be a good idea to delay her invitation to "help" until after your nursing career is well underway. At the very least, counterbalance her negative attitude by including some strong advocates in your support group.

Available. You may have found a very knowledgeable and supportive lactation consultant, but if you can't reach her when your breasts feel like they are going to explode and your new baby has been screaming for two hours, she won't be much help. When you are interviewing pediatricians, lactation consultants, and nurses, make sure you ask them, "How do I reach you on Saturday evening if I am having trouble?" They should be able to give you a concrete explanation of their coverage system. You may want to interview one of their backup people to make sure that you will feel comfortable with *their* advice as well.

Availability is extremely important the first few days after you get home. If you can't talk to someone in your support group when problems arise at 2 A.M., you may be tempted to reach for a bottle of formula. This could be the beginning of the end of a nursing experience that might have been rescued by some timely advice and encouragement. After the second week your questions about scheduling or your diet can wait a day or two (the time it takes for some people to answer their voice mail), but in that first week you need on-call advice twenty-four hours a day.

Experienced. Be sure to ask how long the so-called expert you're consulting has been giving advice. Have they or their partners breastfed their children? How did it go? Don't discard someone from your short list because they don't have much experience, but make sure you also include someone with gray hair who has "been around for awhile."

Flexible and realistic. Some of the most knowledgeable advocates of breastfeeding you meet may lack the ability to adapt to the realities of your unique situation. They may not share my view that you can have a very positive nursing experience that lasts for "only" three months. They may harp on the importance of breastfeeding and miss the point that how you nourish your baby is just one aspect of parenting.

To get a feel for how realistic and flexible they can be, ask your potential advisors some questions. "I plan on weaning when I go back to work after three months. How should I do that?" Or, "Do you ever recommend formula to mothers who are breastfeeding?" Their answers may reveal a bias against your three-month plan.

THE USUAL SUSPECTS

Your obstetrician. Although you might assume that because of your obstetrician's interest in your pregnancy and the health of your fetus/child, that he or she would be a logical choice for your support group, think again. One survey of obstetricians in training revealed that less than 40 percent of them recalled receiving any formal instruction in breastfeeding.

The more dramatic life-and-death events that surround the birth of your baby understandably push less urgent issues such as breastfeeding into the background. Unfortunately, they seldom reemerge in the minds of most obstetricians. Midwives are often more tuned in to the importance of getting nursing off to a good start. That doesn't mean that you shouldn't discuss breastfeeding with your obstetrician. If she has breastfed her children, ask about her own experiences. If your obstetrician is male, ask if his wife nursed their children. How did it go? You may discover that your obstetrician is the exception . . . not only very interested in breastfeeding but with practical experience under her belt.

The pediatrician. While on average pediatricians receive more training about breastfeeding than obstetricians, most of this is in a lecture format. That is, they may have little practical experience. In one survey only about 60 percent of practicing physicians knew that introducing formula in the first few weeks of life was likely to sabotage breastfeeding. It is troubling that so many doctors are unaware of this potential misstep.

That said, almost every pediatrician realizes that breastfeeding is the best way to feed babies, and your baby's doctor should be included in your support group. When you are interviewing pediatricians ask about their commitment to and knowledge about nursing. Did they or their spouse nurse? Personal experience is usually a good indicator of commitment and competence. What is their availability? Who will you be talking to after hours? This will be important not only for questions about breastfeeding but also when your child is sick.

Ask other parents how the pediatrician handled their questions about nursing. Was he or she supportive, knowledgeable, and available? There are some very good pediatricians who aren't terribly knowledgeable about breastfeeding. If you have found a physician whom you like but whom you suspect won't be much help with nursing, consider adding a knowledgeable lactation consultant to your support group.

A lactation consultant. In the last few years many hospitals have been adding lactation consultants to their staffs, although many of these women work independently from their homes. While most lactation consultants have taken courses about breastfeeding and have passed certification exams, this does not guarantee that you will feel comfortable working with just any certified lactation consultant. Nursing is a very personal experience, and you should carefully interview consultants. Ask friends for recommendations.

I have found that lactation consultants can be extremely helpful in the first week of nursing, when difficulties with attachment are the most critical. An experienced lactation consultant can often rescue a nursing situation that is faltering because of faulty attachment by offering advice and providing hands-on adjustments.

On the other hand, some lactation consultants are so focused on the value of breastfeeding that they lose sight of the realities of your life, like the fact that you're going back to work in a few months. They may unintentionally make you feel guilty because you have decided that you aren't going to nurse for a year or even six months. Breastfeeding may have come easily for them, and they may have trouble understanding why you aren't enjoying nursing as much as they did.

Remember, one of the reasons that I have written this book is to help women like yourself enjoy nursing on their own terms. Your lactation consultant may not agree with some of my advice, particularly when it comes to fostering sleep independence. This is an honest difference of opinion. It doesn't mean that either one of us is wrong. You can take their advice about attachment and sore nipples, and follow my suggestions about scheduling and weaning, for instance. In fact, you may find that you will have the most satisfying nursing experience by combining advice from several sources. No one of us has all the right answers.

Family members. While you may be envious of women who can look to their families as a knowledgeable and available nursing support group, you aren't alone. I suspect that most women your age don't have a family member experienced in breastfeeding living close by.

It may comfort you to learn that after analyzing some data collected in the 1980s, researchers could find no evidence that having available family members had a positive effect on a young mother's pre- or postnatal health. In fact they found that "closer kin access is associated with a *lower* probability of breastfeeding."[*]

In other words, you might want to think twice before including family members in your support group. They may in fact make it more difficult for you to get breastfeeding well established. This might surprise you, because it has become traditional to invite one or both grandmothers to come "help" in the first few weeks. However, I have seen many unfortunate situations in

---

[*]L. M. Casper et al., "Family Networks in Prenatal and Postnatal Health," *Social Biology*, vol. 37 (1–2), pp. 84–101, 1994.

which a well-meaning grandmother or an aunt has unintentionally sabotaged a new mother's attempts at nursing by an ill-timed or poorly managed visit.

Now, before you call the AARP and report me as an anti-American, apple pie–hating grandmother-basher, let me explain. First, you will soon learn that sleep, both for you and your baby, is an important ingredient in the mix that can make or break your breastfeeding experience. After the first few days, it will be very helpful to have your baby sleeping in his own room. If, like most young families, you don't have a bedroom to spare, you may be tempted to offer Grandmother a bed in the nursery, and keep the baby in your bedroom. While this arrangement may work for the first week, it will eventually interfere with the important process of "settling in." Interrupted and poor quality sleep for both you and the baby will result in fatigue, one of the most potent poisons to breastfeeding. In other words, grandmothers' visits should not displace anyone from their usual sleeping place.

Fortunately, I encounter very few grandmothers who are outwardly negative about nursing. However, many of them lack practical experience and enough confidence in the value of breastfeeding to provide reassurance that can be critical to a worried new mother having second thoughts during those first difficult days. Misguided advice about pacifiers and schedules can interfere with the process of getting the milk established, and panicky suggestions to offer formula at the wrong time may send breastfeeding into a tailspin from which it cannot recover.

How should you handle this dilemma? You know that inviting her or both grandmothers is the polite and traditional thing to do. While you suspect that she will be supportive, you certainly don't want her presence to interfere with your efforts. Let me be the bad guy, and offer some suggestions that may be helpful.

First, make sure that your "helper" has a place to sleep that will allow you and your baby to remain in your own rooms and in your own beds. If you don't have a spare bedroom, offer to help Grandma find a nearby motel or a room with a friend or neighbor. Create a list of chores and errands that she can work her way through. This is particularly helpful if she doesn't know much about breastfeeding. Retain the hands-on-baby things for yourself. Even changing diapers will be fun for the first few days. Each opening will bring a new "surprise." She can be responsible for cooking, laundry, shopping, and housecleaning. Her payment will come in the form of holding the baby from time to time, but be careful not to allow overhandling by someone other than yourself. It can make some babies cranky.

If you are concerned that your mother may erode your confidence because she is a worrier, ask her to help out after you have gotten the nursing well underway. This will usually take about two weeks, and will hopefully coincide with your husband's return to work.

Although you may love your mother dearly, you and she may have the kind of relationship that casts you as the hostess whenever she comes to visit. This may mean that even though you have a temperature of 104°F, you feel obliged to fix her a five-course gourmet meal. If this sounds familiar, delay your mother's visit until your baby is at least a month old. Unless you can escape your role as chef-chambermaid-concierge, you will be just too exhausted in the first few months to entertain your mother, or any other guest, for that matter. It might be a good idea to talk about the first visit with your mom now. I'll bet that she will gladly allow you to drop your Martha Stewart imitation in exchange for the chance to see her newly born grandchild.

Your husband. Unless your husband was previously married and had helped his first wife with breastfeeding, we probably can't count him being either an experienced or knowledgeable member of your support group. Nonetheless, his presence on the team as a cheerleader, spokesperson, and go-fer is extremely important.

It will be difficult for you to sustain your enthusiasm for breastfeeding if your husband is not supportive of the idea. In one study when fathers strongly approved of nursing, 98 percent of the women breastfed their newborns. However, if he was indifferent to the feeding choice, only slightly more than 25 percent of the mothers breastfed.* If you can't get your husband to read this book, make sure that you read Chapter 10, "Your Husband's Role in the Plan," carefully. It will give you some ideas on how to include him in the process.

Making sense out of conflicting advice. Everyone has his or her own ideas of how breastfeeding is best established and practiced. There are many ways to nurse successfully, and of course there are at least an equal number of ways to get it wrong. Obviously, conflicting advice can be confusing and unsettling, particularly if you are tired, sore, and more than a little bit scared.

Even if you have a lactation consultant as your primary resource for information, you will still rely on several other people for emotional and logistical support. You can count on them to offer advice, even when you haven't asked for it.

Accept the inevitability of conflicting advice. However, you can minimize the conflict by providing your advisers with as much information as you can before you ask your question. Don't let them fall into the trap of giving you bad advice because they don't have all the facts. For example, breastfeeding infants who are older than four weeks of age will often skip three or four days between bowel movements. This is perfectly normal. However, if your two-week-old hasn't had a bowel movement in three days, something is probably wrong. If your adviser doesn't know exactly how old your baby is, he or she may reassure you that everything is fine when the better advice would be to bring in the child for an evaluation.

Of course if you get dramatically different answers from two different people, ask a third and fourth and so on until you are comfortable that you have a consensus. Remember that there are many correct ways to nurse. I hope with the help of this book and the advice of others, you will develop a unique nursing style that works best for you.

---

*H. Littman et al., "The Decision to Breastfeed: The Importance of Father's Approval," *Clinical Pediatrics,* vol. 33(4), pp. 214–19, 1994.

FINDING A BREASTFEEDING-FRIENDLY HOSPITAL

The first few days can be extremely important to your breastfeeding success. Hospital policies and the attitude and experience of the nursing staff can either promote nursing or lead to a premature termination. In 1991 the World Health Organization (WHO) and UNICEF acknowledged this critical role of hospitals by launching the Baby-Friendly Hospital Initiative. Hospitals receiving the designation of "Baby-Friendly" must demonstrate that their policies promote breastfeeding. While a total of 6,000 hospitals worldwide have been designated "Baby-Friendly," as of 1996 only 309 hospitals in the United States had received "Certificates of Intent" to seek this designation. Only a single U.S. hospital had completed the process.

In other words, don't assume that hospital care carries a guaranteed nursing-friendly environment. One survey of health professionals taken in North Carolina in 1993 found that pediatricians and nutritionists had the most positive beliefs about nursing, but hospital nurses (who provide the bulk of hands-on patient care) were more likely to have negative beliefs about breastfeeding.* Another study done at a hospital in Arizona reported that mothers who were discharged early nursed longer. While that observation is atypical, it does suggest that some hospitals may have such a negative impact on breastfeeding that mothers may be better off at home.

If you have a choice of hospitals, make one or two visits before your delivery and interview their staffs to help you decide which hospital is more supportive of nursing. Here are some questions to ask and the answers to look for (for more about the importance of the answers, see Chapters 11, 12, and 13):

- <u>Will I be able to nurse in the delivery room?</u> "Yes, usually you will be able to breastfeed your baby within five or ten minutes after birth."

* E. Barnett et al., *Birth*, vol. 22(1) (1995), pp. 15–20.

- <u>Will my baby be able to stay in my room with me?</u> "Yes, and we will be encouraging you to nurse him as often as he seems hungry, even if that means every hour for awhile."

- <u>Will you offer my baby a pacifier?</u> "No, we know it interferes with breastfeeding."

- <u>Will you offer my baby sugar water?</u> "Yes, but only if his blood sugar is low and has stayed low after you have nursed him. Occasionally, we will give him sugar water if the doctor thinks your baby is dehydrated, but we always try to use a syringe and tube and not a nipple."

- <u>Have you breastfed your own children? What about the other nurses?</u> "Yes, I did, and most of the other nurses have as well."

- <u>Is there a lactation consultant on the staff? How often does she make rounds?</u> "Yes, and she or her partner come around everyday, but we also expect you to ring for one of us whenever you need help with nursing."

If you don't have a choice of hospitals, you should still make a visit and ask these questions. If the answers suggest that the hospital may not be nursing-friendly, broach the subject with your obstetrician and pediatrician. Ask them to help you by writing orders in your hospital charts (yours and your baby's) that will help the nursing staff create an atmosphere that is more conducive to breastfeeding. For example, the pediatrician can order that your baby not receive a pacifier or a sugar water bottle unless both you and the pediatrician have been consulted. She can also arrange for a rooming-in situation. The obstetrician can see that you are given the chance to feed your baby in the delivery room. These are not unreasonable requests, but the fact that you must make them is a sad commentary on the medical community's ignorance and lack of commitment to breastfeeding.

CLEARING YOUR CALENDAR

Whether you breastfeed or not, the birth of your baby will change your life forever. You must first accept and then learn to play by a new set of rules. Becoming a parent means that another life has been inserted into the space that you have been occupying by yourself since you were born.

You might be thinking, "I've already been there, done that. I have been sharing my life with my husband since we got married." The few adjustments you have made in your life to accommodate your spouse are trivial compared to those to come. Some activities have become so tightly woven into your schedule that you may not be able to differentiate between those that are truly essential and those that you'll dispense with when your baby arrives. Reading the paper, doing the crossword puzzle, exercising in the morning, and going out to dinner and a movie are just a few examples of activities that may temporarily disappear with the arrival of your child. Some of them may be gone forever.

Please listen to those of us with children. Taking care of your baby is so consuming and exhausting that for a while you'll be working hard to make time for a shower, let alone a movie. Begin by clearing your calendar for at least the first two months after delivery. That means no meetings, no appointments (other than trips to the pediatrician and obstetrician), no family reunions, no bridal showers or weddings. If your sister is getting married in the first couple of months after your delivery and asks you to be an attendant, I urge you to respectfully (and perhaps tearfully) decline. If you simply can't refuse, at least give yourself an out, explaining that you can't anticipate what shape you and the baby will be in. Tell her that your level of participation will be on a "can do" basis, and make it clear that if you have gotten off to a shaky start with motherhood, you may be forced to assume the spectator role.

Don't agree to "just a little part-time" work at home. It is never as little work as you or your boss anticipated. I can guarantee that parenting is a full-time job; during the first couple of months it is more like one and a half jobs. This may be difficult if, like me, you are a workaholic. However, even those of us who are energized by our work find that parenthood is more than enough challenge to keep us stimulated . . . at least for the first couple of months.

As you begin to feel comfortable with motherhood and as breastfeeding becomes well established, you will begin to rebuild your life with your baby's needs in mind. Chapter 20 will give you some suggestions about what activities you might want to add gradually. There is life after delivery and there is life while you are breastfeeding. It's best to start with a clean slate.

PROTECTING YOUR PRIVACY

There is nothing that draws a crowd faster than a new baby. I can guarantee that you will get more phone calls and more visitors than you could possibly want. Some will ask if you need help, but everyone will be curious to see what this new addition to the family looks like.

That's all well and good, but you need time to sleep and feed your baby. There just aren't enough hours in the day for you to breastfeed and entertain all of your friends and relatives during those first exhausting weeks. This is particularly true if, like many women, you feel uncomfortable nursing in public or even among close family and friends.

Initially there may be as many as ten or twelve feedings each day, and your novice status means they will be time-consuming. (Two months down the road you'll reduce feeding time by half.) To conserve your energy and repay your sleep debt from night feedings, you will be napping when your baby does.

If you are going to make breastfeeding work and be rested enough to enjoy the experience, you will need to erect some barriers to protect your privacy. I know that it can be difficult to discourage your family and friends from visiting, but limiting these visits is essential. By all means make me the bad guy if you think it will make things go more smoothly. I don't mind.

Dad can, and should, take a lead role in protecting you from the curious hordes. He can become the doorman, the press secretary, and the bouncer, depending on the situation. Tell him not to be afraid to turn away uninvited visitors by telling them that you are sleeping or nursing the baby. Work out a signal that will alert him that you are getting tired and it is time to usher the invited guests out the door.

Make sure that your answering machine is working and turn down the ringer. Update your message often, so those who get the machine experience the next best thing to getting you. For example, "Baby Emily is feeding well, fifteen minutes on each side. She has pooped twice and pee'd three times since the last update. Mother Marjorie is still a bit tired, but is feeling well. Leave a message if you like and we will try to get back to you between naps and feedings. Call for the next Emily Update at three this afternoon." Of course if you have created a website for your baby, this can be kept current with details and even digital pictures.

Eventually you will be ready to entertain and show off your new baby, but during those first few weeks, every hour you can keep for yourself for feeding and sleeping will pay huge dividends. Don't be afraid to appear a bit rude or antisocial. The parents who remember what it was like will understand, and those who don't will soon forget that you didn't invite them in or return every call.

FINDING A NURSING-FRIENDLY DAYCARE OPTION

If you hope to continue breastfeeding when you return to work, you'll need daycare that compliments and encourages nursing. Good daycare is hard to come by under any circumstances, and adding the additional condition that it should be nursing-friendly ups the ante. That's why it's important to start before your baby arrives. Let's look at some of the factors you should consider as you evaluate your options.

Overall quality. Whether you decide to continue breastfeeding or not, you want your child to be cared for by people who know what they are doing and do it well. There is nothing more distracting for a mother than to worry that her child is anything less than comfortable, safe, and appropriately stimulated. Yes, breastfeeding is important, but don't sacrifice quality in your daycare selection simply because you have found an environment that you think will be more nursing-friendly. Fortunately, this is seldom the problem. You can usually count on most daycare providers that support breastfeeding to provide quality care.

Attitude. Your child's daycare provider can be an important member of your nursing support group. If she understands how important nursing is to your family, you can count on her as a shoulder to lean on when you are having a bad nursing day. Hopefully she can bend some rules and schedules to ease your transition back to work. For example, if you had planned to run over to the daycare at ten to nurse your baby, but he wakes hungry at nine-thirty, that next half hour could be rather unpleasant. If your daycare provider is supportive of your efforts to breastfeed, she may spend the time entertaining your child instead of reaching for a bottle of formula just to quiet him down. She realizes that by giving that bottle she could interrupt the natural rhythm of supply and demand between you and your baby.

As you interview potential daycare providers, ask them how they feel about breastfeeding. Did they nurse their babies? Present the scenario I have just described. How would they handle it?

Experience. Has the daycare you are considering had much experience with mothers who hope to continue breastfeeding when they return to work? Do they understand that babies who are fed breast milk may need to feed more often? Can they build some flexibility into their schedules? Have they endured those difficult situations when a baby who has never taken a bottle is separated from his mother for six or eight hours? The experienced daycare provider has been there many times, so she won't call you at work in a panic to tell you that your baby hasn't had anything to drink in four hours. She knows that eventually thirst will overcome his stubborn streak.

Proximity. The most nursing-friendly daycare is one that is a five-minute walk from your office. This proximity will allow you to zip over for a quick half-hour feeding several times during the day. Some enlightened businesses provide in-house daycare because they realize that it actually increases the productivity of their employees, but the truth is these arrangements are difficult to find.

Close proximity is most critical in the first six months. After that, nursings will be more widely spaced and replaced by solid food. Keep this in mind as you are choosing a daycare. The daycare you select for the first six to twelve months doesn't need to offer recreational space or stress social interaction with peers. In fact it is healthier for your infant to avoid large numbers of small children. After his first birthday, when you won't need to be there for breastfeeding, you can move your child to a different, perhaps more distant site that offers a more physically stimulating environment.

A space to nurse and/or pump. Unless you live very close to the daycare, you and your baby will probably want to nurse just before you separate and as soon as you see each other again. Does the daycare offer a place where you can do so in comfort and privacy?

CREATING A NURSING-FRIENDLY WORKPLACE

Now is the time! Your pregnancy may leave you feeling drained at the end of the day, but motherhood, whether or not you breastfeed, will be even more exhausting. Take advantage of what time and energy you have left to evaluate your workplace and make what nursing-friendly modifications you can.

Some of the rearrangements may require structural changes such as hanging doors, moving cubicles, and painting walls. Others may involve disrupting schedules and vacations. These things take time. Your employer and fellow workers may be much more cooperative if you have given them advance warning of your intentions to continue nursing after you return to work.

Assemble your allies. Network with fellow workers who have breastfed. Find out what worked and what didn't. If you will be the first woman in your office to return to work while she is still breastfeeding, you will be venturing into uncharted territory. You will certainly have to do some educating and advocating. You may have to look beyond your own department for support. Talk to other women with child-bearing potential. In a few months or years they may be beneficiaries of your efforts to create a nursing-friendly workplace. Look for support wherever you can find it. For example, if your boss is a man, talk to his wife, a potentially persuasive and powerful ally, at the Christmas party or the annual picnic.

Unfortunately, you won't have our judicial system on your side. So far attempts to treat breastfeeding as a disabling condition that deserves special legal protection under the Pregnancy Discrimination Act of 1978 have been generally unsuccessful. If you live in Minnesota, a 1998 law says that your employer must provide you with "reasonable unpaid breaktime" to express milk and must provide you with a private space for pumping. However, it is unlikely that Congress will enact similar nursing-friendly legislation for the rest of us any time in the near future.

Without support from the government, you must convince your employer that creating a breastfeeding-friendly workplace is not only the right thing to do but also the profitable thing to do. One researcher has found that women who breastfed their infants had 30 percent less absenteeism due to their children's illnesses. The insurance company CIGNA has recently implemented a lactation program and found that after four years mothers enrolled in the program had 77 percent less absenteeism compared to other new mothers and were saving the company $300,000 per year in health costs. Unfortunately, this is one of the only examples you can currently cite to your employer. However, I am sure that over the next few years other enlightened companies will be publicizing the profitability they have enjoyed by creating breastfeeding-friendly workplaces.

Take all of your maternity leave . . . and then some. All of the data that I have seen clearly show that the longer you can stay at home, the more likely you will be able to continue to breastfeed once you do return to work. It takes most women at least six weeks to really get the hang of breastfeeding and to begin to get enough rest to recover from their delivery. If you return to work at eight weeks, you may have had only two weeks to really enjoy breast-feeding.

The more firmly nursing has become established, the more resistant it will be to the negative pressures that are an inevitable part of going back to work. With time, ten or twelve feedings per day will become five or six. Three or four night wakings will decrease to one . . . or less.

I view twelve weeks as a minimum maternity leave if you hope to continue breastfeeding when you return to work. Four months should be your target, or at least an initial negotiating point. Obviously, six months is even better. However, I have written this book for mothers who are living and working in the real world, and you are probably going to have trouble getting even nine weeks. This is another reason to start your planning as soon as possible. There may be personal and vacation days that you can bank and apply to your maternity leave. Open the negotiations now. It will take time to arrange an extended maternity leave.

While statistics show that women who go back to work part-time usually nurse longer than those who return full-time, resist the offers of part-time work before eight weeks. I have seen mothers fall into this trap too often. Part-time work always expands into a bigger commitment than you or your employer planned, and you will be more fatigued by your delivery than you expected.

If at all possible plan a slow return to full-time work that stretches over a month or two. While you must consider your own unique job schedule and commuting arrangement as you are planning your return to work, I have a few suggestions based on my observation of several thousand nursing mothers. First, five short office days is usually better than three long days in the office and two off. Your body and your baby will appreciate the predictability of five similar days. Long days will usually mean less nursing and more pumping. Your body may respond to this on-again-off-again arrangement by making less milk.

Second, a part-time schedule that allows you to arrive late and leave early has several advantages. You will find that getting organized and out of the house in the morning takes a lot more time when you have a baby. In addition, the first nursing of the day is usually a more substantial feeding and hence takes more time. This kind of schedule often has the added advantage of requiring a shorter commute time because you won't be traveling during rush hour.

Your creativity and time management skills will be rewarded with a longer and/or more enjoyable nursing experience. While you can't predict exactly how your schedule will work out, start making *realistic* plans now. Explore arrangements such as job sharing and flex-time. If you've been a valuable employee, you may be pleasantly surprised how accommodating your employer and fellow workers may be.

Establish when and where to pump. Unless you have been able to find a daycare across the street from your office, you are going to have to pump your breasts to maintain your milk supply. While many mothers are comfortable nursing their baby in the presence of strangers, I have yet to meet a woman who pumps her breasts in public. It just doesn't work.

You will need to find a place that is clean, comfortable, and private to pump. In the past many women were offered the public rest room. This is *not* an acceptable solution. Don't even allow it on the negotiating table. For starters, it isn't really private and it probably isn't terribly clean or comfortable either.

You will need a room with a door that latches, a comfortable chair, and an electric socket for the pump. If you are fortunate enough to have your own office, you may not need to look any further. However, many modern offices have glass walls or are little more than a cubicle, so privacy may be a problem. Begin your hunt for space now. Are there storage rooms that you could offer to clean out and redecorate? Are there co-workers who would be willing to trade space for a few months? Although it is hard to predict exactly what your pumping schedule will be, you can safely estimate that you will need the room for two or, at most, three half-hour sessions each eight-hour workday.

Of course your employer must be willing to grant you this time. Resist the offer to use your entire lunch break for pumping. Eating is a separate activity, and although you may be able to snack while you are pumping, you should request additional time for pumping. Start now to arrange coverage of your duties. Remember, good preparation is your best defense against the unpredictability of biologic processes like breastfeeding.

You will also need access to a refrigerator to store your breast milk. If it is going to be fed to your baby within twenty-four hours, simple refrigeration is fine. If you are planning on saving it any longer, you will need a good freezer. OSHA (Occupational Safety and Health Administration) regulations about use of refrigerators are strict. You won't be able to store breastmilk in a refrigerator that is intended for medical supplies or chemicals. However, the one in the lunchroom is fine.

Even if you manage to juggle schedules, negotiate time-off, and find an acceptable pumping room before your return to work, there will be challenges the first day back—separation from your baby for the first time, fatigue, and the less-than-supportive attitude of some of your co-workers, to name just a few. Chapter 21, "The Third Month," will address these and other hurdles you may have to clear when you return to work.

THE HOME-OFFICE OPTION: HOME BUT NOT ALONE

Perhaps you're one of an increasing number of women who work out of their homes. What could be better? You'll nurse him when he is hungry and still get your work done. No commutes, no daycare hassles, no pumping. Sounds perfect, doesn't it? Not quite. While you've avoided many of the challenges, there is some downside.

Take, for example, Kate's experience. She is a medical transcriptionist who with a computer and a fax machine hoped to continue her work from home after her baby was born. At her baby's two-month checkup, Kate tearfully told me that it wasn't working. Halfway through transcribing a medical summary her baby would start crying, and she would stop to feed him. After feeding for ten minutes he'd fall asleep. She would put him down and perhaps work for fifteen minutes before he started crying again. The doctors she worked for were complaining about errors in her work, and she was staying up late to meet her deadlines. She started off each day exhausted.

Kate erroneously assumed that because she would be at home she didn't need to create a schedule or routine for the baby. In fact, 24/7 access to her baby was something she considered a big plus about working at home. However, the sword cut both ways. Without a set schedule, her baby came to expect her breast whenever things weren't going his way. Kate had become a pacifier.

Watching scores of mothers experiment with the working at home, it's obvious that the most successful among them created a routine and set limits that allowed them to get their job done as well as reap the benefits of being near their baby. No one's perfect and even with a schedule, you'll face unexpected challenges . . . but nothing like the stress Kate felt.

The truth is that for the first month (or two) you can't expect to keep a regular schedule. Your baby's feeding pattern will simply be unpredictable, so you shouldn't count on getting much work done. However, if you follow the suggestions in chapters 20 and 21 about sleep management and building a routine, you eventually should be able to schedule several two-hour work periods throughout the day. But it can't happen if you have allowed yourself to become your child's pacifier.

It is also important to create some physical separation between your work space and the rest of your home, particularly if you plan to continue working at home for your child's first few years. Rosemary is a bookkeeper who was able to retain most of her clients and stay at home with her baby. She kept a Port-a-Crib and eventually a small playpen in the small office/study she and her husband had built off the back of their family room. Initially the arrangement was very convenient; she could nurse her baby and keep an eye on him, too. However, it limited her ability to use her printer and fax machine because the noise often woke the baby. Once mobile, her son continually threatened to wreak havoc, and on one occasion almost deleted a large payroll account by turning off the computer. Even after she hired a high school student to come in after school to entertain him, he regularly wandered into her office and interrupted what she was doing.

By defining her office as off-limits to her baby from the time the baby arrived at home, she could have avoided most of the interruptions that followed. While initially it may seem rather arbitrary to keep your baby's crib in another room, it is a signal to him (and a reminder to you) that there is a separation between your job and mothering. As Kate's experience demonstrates, you're going to need chunks of uninterrupted time to get anything done.

If you establish a separation from the beginning, your child is less likely to challenge the office as off-limits rule because he has never known it could be any different. Of course as your child gets older (sometime in the second six months) you may need to employ someone to entertain him and help with the household chores. This will depend on how many hours your job demands and how flexible your work schedule can be. However, even if your hours are flexible, I think that it will be less confusing for your child if you create a consistent routine. Children love and understand routines. It will be much easier for you to say that you will play with him "after his nap" or "after *Mister Rogers*'" instead of "later," which is too open-ended to satisfy most youngsters.

I know a lawyer who worked at home until her daughter was two. By the time her child was eight months old, she had created an established routine. She would leave the house by the front door when the sitter arrived, walk around to the side door, and go into her office in the rear of the house. She would then "return" again through the front door at noon for a lunch break. Initially, the child was unaware that her mother was still in the house! Eventually the child wised up, but felt no temptation to interrupt her mother's work, because that part of the house had always been off-limits during office hours. While this charade may seem silly to you, there's no doubt it was successful and demonstrates that setting some simple limits can make all the difference.

BUY A BREAST PUMP

You may have decided that you will wean your baby when your maternity leave is over and so won't need a breast pump. But you will! A breast pump can be a valuable weapon in your battle against engorgement and fatigue during those first critical days. At two in the morning of your first night home, your husband won't find one on the shelves at the local convenience store—so shop for and buy a breast pump when you have the time.

Manual pumps can be purchased for as little as $20, but most women find these difficult to operate and inefficient. At the other end of the spectrum are electric models made by Medela, which can pump both of your breasts simultaneously and have a refrigerated storage compartment. If you have already decided to continue nursing when you return to work, their cost (several hundred dollars) may be easily repaid by their efficiency. Renting a pump from the hospital or lactation consultant is another option. Ask your insurance company and employer if they will cover some, or all, of the expense.

The Isis by Avent has received five-star reviews from mothers for its ease of operation and breast-friendly design. Its $40 price tag makes it an excellent choice for moms on a budget. Although it is hand operated, many women have found the Isis continues to meet their needs when they return to work.

While you will be the one using the pump, ask your mechanically inclined husband to help you in its selection. All pumps require cleaning and reassembly, and he may enjoy being your one-man pit crew.

10

Your Husband's Role
in the Plan

When you imagine nursing, what do you see? If you're like most
of the women I see in my office, you visualize a woman with a
contented smile on her face, enjoying a special moment with her
child. But wait. Someone is missing. Where is the father? What is
he doing while his wife and child share this unique nutritional
and emotional experience?

Breastfeeding advocates, psychologists, physicians, nurses, and
lactation consultants have given very little attention to a father's
contribution to breastfeeding. This oversight is unfortunate
because a husband can play, and in many cases must play, a critical role in his wife's nursing experience. If your Maternity Leave
Breastfeeding Plan is going to work, you need your husband or
partner as a contributing member of your support group. His role
is that of advocate, cheerleader, and helper, willing to share
enough of the hard work of parenting to help you stay well rested.
If your plan includes returning to work, his assistance is
absolutely essential.

When the two of you discussed breastfeeding six months prior
to the delivery date, your husband may have sounded like one of
your strongest supporters. When the baby arrives, you will both
be faced with the fact that being the father of a nursing baby may
not turn out to be as wonderful as you expected. This discrepancy
between expectations and realities can create an ambivalence
about breastfeeding that undermines his support. Understanding
these feelings will help you reassure him while he struggles with

what it means to be a father. Ironically, there may be a few days when you have to prop up the person you were counting on to be your biggest supporter.

Like many men your husband may find the role of bystander frustrating. After months of planning and sharing the pregnancy, attending Lamaze classes together, and coaching you through labor, maybe even cutting the cord, he is suddenly on the sidelines because he is not biologically equipped for the next great adventure.

As the father of three children I can tell you that I had some very unrealistic expectations about parenthood. I anticipated cuddling my new baby and playing with her for hours at time. She would look at me and smile. If there was a problem, I could comfort and protect her. It was going to be fun, and I would be busy doing things for her, making sure that she was growing up strong and healthy. Reality was very different. Initially, she was either sleeping or eating, and I couldn't feed her because, well, because I couldn't feed her. I could hold her briefly, but she quickly got tired, hungry, or upset, which meant putting her down or giving her to my wife to nurse. Her mother could calm her and make things better. Her mother was the one who was making sure that she was growing up big and strong. It was disappointing and frustrating. It was like being stood up for a date. I was all dressed up and had nothing to do. I could see it was going to be a great party, and I didn't have a date. My wife and my daughter were having all the fun, and I was sitting out every dance.

Your husband will probably feel many of the same things. The few scientific studies that have been done reveal that most fathers feel like outsiders when their children are being nursed. This new nonrole can be very damaging to a father's self-esteem. All of us like to feel needed, and for the moment biology has assigned you, the mother, the primary parenting role. Breastfeeding can also contribute to feelings of inadequacy that may have plagued your husband before the baby was born. He may have waited patiently through your pregnancy hoping that once you delivered there would be more for him to do.

For some new fathers this bystander role is merely disappointing; for others it's depressing or frustrating. Most dads keep these emotions hidden. Rationally, they know what's best for their babies. However, some of his formerly positive feelings may be replaced by negative ones as he realizes that he is being left out of the loop. Don't worry, as the weeks go by there will be more and more opportunities for him to get involved.

Fortunately, most fathers deal successfully with the biologic reality that they can't breastfeed by employing what some psychologists term postponement. The father of a nursing baby has no choice but to postpone many of the rewards of fatherhood until breastfeeding is no longer the primary activity of his child's day. You and I can help him by laying out a realistic timetable of activities and events he can be a part of.

WHAT A FATHER *CAN* DO . . .

Change diapers. I always enjoy watching new parents learn to diaper their baby. There are never enough hands, but plenty of bodily fluids to go around. For the parents of a breastfed baby a diaper change is (initially) a kind of validation. Each wet or messy diaper is a piece of evidence that breastfeeding is working. If something is coming out, there must be something going in! And it doesn't smell!

If your husband avoids diaper changing like the plague, don't press him, but I suspect he will be thrilled at the opportunity to handle his baby and survey the by-products of his wife's efforts. After a month or two changing diapers loses its charm for even the most enthusiastic parent, but in the beginning it can and should be a way to involve Dad in babycare.

Burp the baby. If your husband is around at feeding times, make Dad the designated burper. Some fathers become more adept at this skill than their wives. For each feeding there are potentially four opportunities to burp the baby. Remember to limit each burping attempt to two or three minutes. If a burp doesn't come up right away, it probably isn't going to come up in the near future. Dragging the process out is only going to tire or annoy the baby, or both. Sit side by side on the couch and pass the baby back and forth as each of you does your thing.

Protect you and your baby from your adoring fans. Newborn babies attract visitors like bears to honey—every one of them wanting to see, touch, and hold this new addition to the clan, and they're oblivious to your fatigue and desire for privacy while you nurse.

Intrusions upon the innermost workings of your newly created family can interfere with breastfeeding unless someone steps in to shield you and your baby from at least some of the attention. Your husband is the best choice for this role of protector, press agent, and bouncer. Ask him to answer the phone and tell callers when you are resting or nursing. He can give short progress reports and assure loved ones that you'll call back later when you are feeling up to it.

Your husband should be the one to answer the door and receive gifts, turning away those who have not called ahead, screening small children for signs of illness, and reminding everyone he allows in that the baby may need to nurse at any time, in which case they may be asked to leave. If visitors overstay their welcome, he can fabricate an excuse and ask them to leave.

This job of bouncer is not easy. It demands some assertiveness and a flair for tactfulness, but it is important if you and your baby are going to get enough rest to make the Maternity Leave Breastfeeding Plan work.

Bathe. While I suggest that parents give their babies a submersion bath just two or three times per week in the winter, to avoid seasonal dry skin, your baby should be sponge bathed daily. This is an excellent opportunity for Dad to step in and take charge. Before you get the hang of it the process will probably take two of you.

Two warnings about bathing. First, babies are distinctly divided into two camps: those who love their baths and those who hate them. If your baby is a card-carrying member of the latter group, you might reconsider Dad's role as bath master general. Our goal here is to create a positive interaction between a father and his baby. If on the contrary your baby screams from bath start to finish, you might want to retain that duty for yourself.

Second, baths can overstimulate some babies, while for others the process may be very soothing. If your husband can help out only in the evenings and your baby is jazzed up by his bath, it may be better for all concerned to have you give the bath early in the day. Your baby's sleep is more important than who gives him the bath. A wet and wild event late in the day is very likely to interfere with the your baby's settling into a good sleep pattern.

Dress. Here is another very physical activity for your husband to take a stab at. One of my perverse pleasures is watching new parents redress a newborn in full winter regalia after a visit in my office. It can take forever, and unfortunately I seldom have the time to observe the entire event. There are arms, legs, snaps, zippers, drawstrings, and Velcro everywhere. Babies aren't as fragile as they look, but new parents are invariably cautious as they insert each extremity into the appropriate (or at times inappropriate) opening of garment after garment. Offering your husband the chance to participate in these sartorial wrestling matches can provide him ten or fifteen minutes of together time per dressing.

Hold the baby. Even though your husband can't nurse his new baby there is nothing to prevent him from holding the baby and enjoying some of the tactile pleasures of parenthood . . . well, almost nothing. The problem is that for the first month your baby pretty much just eats and sleeps. This doesn't leave very much time for recreational holding by anyone . . . you, your husband, Grandmother, Aunt Louise, whomever. There may be little snatches of time, ten to fifteen minutes in length, after daytime feedings. However, you must be careful. If you want your baby to develop good sleep habits, it's important he learns to fall asleep exclusively in his own bed. You don't want him nodding off at your breast or in his father's arms. We want your baby to associate the pleasurable experience of drifting off to slumberland with his bed, not your arms or anyone else's lap. If your baby is one who rapidly falls asleep after feedings, this isn't going to leave much of an opportunity for poor Dad to get in much holding time.

Let's try to remain reasonable and flexible here. There are times when it is fine for the new father to allow his baby to fall asleep in his arms. The pleasure your husband derives can outweigh the risk of interfering with your baby's sleep habits. Flexibility, moderation, and compromise are important characteristics of successful family life. As long as your baby seems happy and is sleeping well, your husband can hold the baby as long as he wishes. I am merely reminding you that the development of your baby's sleep habits should be given an extremely high priority and must be balanced against his father's desire to become part of the picture.

Become a technical adviser. If your husband is intrigued by things mechanical, he can take on the role of technical adviser. One facet of nursing that may appeal to his mechanical instincts is the selection and purchase of a breast pump. As there are several options, assign him the task of researching, choosing, and buying the pump. He can then study the directions and become the family expert on cleaning and maintenance. This may be an ongoing project because you may find that despite rave reviews from other mothers, the pump he bought may not be the best choice for you.

While pumping is ultimately your responsibility, your husband can be in charge of storage. Remember, this is an option to offer your husband if he is looking for ways to be helpful. Don't push if these aspects of breastfeeding don't interest him, or if he doesn't view them as meaningful involvement.

Elicit a smile. While many parents claim that their baby smiled from the moment they brought him home, a true social smile doesn't emerge until three to six weeks of age. Seeing one of these first smiles can give Dad strength for the few more months of relative detachment that lie ahead. If your husband is feeling left out, consider "saving" the first smile for him. While you may have observed your baby's first social smile, you might tell your husband that you "thought" that the baby smiled at you but you weren't sure, and then wait the few hours or days it may take before he becomes the recipient of one of these glorious grins. There is nothing wrong with a little white lie now and then, particularly when it helps bring a new dad a bit closer to the center of the family.

Offer a bottle. If your scheduled return to works means that you are going to have to introduce a bottle, your husband can play an important role in the breast-to-bottle transition. This should begin at around four weeks (see Chapter 20). Even if you aren't planning on going back to work, the chance to offer a bottle will give bystander Dad a chance to share in the enjoyment of feeding his baby. Everyone loves to feed babies. The process has powerful magnetism, and once your friends and relatives know that your baby can take a bottle, there will be a waiting list to take a turn. Save the bulk of the feedings for Dad.

I must sound a few notes of caution. First, your baby may resist taking a bottle. It happens. If you are going back to work, you should be patient and persist. However, if you are introducing the bottle merely so that your husband can join in the fun, don't push the issue if it creates an ugly scene. Dad's gratification can be delayed another few weeks when there will be more things for him to do with his baby.

Second, these paternal bottle feedings shouldn't interfere with establishing a good sleeping and eating pattern. Limit them to once a day at most, and make sure that they fit into your baby's day in a manner that is least disruptive to his sleep schedule. Your husband will enjoy these feedings, and he'll want to do as many as you allow. As the months go on, it may work out that he can do two or three a day.

IF YOU PLAN TO GO BACK TO WORK

If your Maternity Leave Breastfeeding Plan isn't the beginning and end of your nursing career, your husband's assistance will be critical to your ongoing success. But even if you wean your baby to formula, you will need all of the help your husband can give.

As I have watched the two-income family evolve over the last two decades, I have been pleasantly surprised by how certain fathers take on traditionally maternal tasks. However, families in which parenting responsibilities are truly divided fifty-fifty are extremely rare. I am not sure that there is much that you or I can do if your husband is one of the clueless who has not accepted the concept of team parenting, but it wouldn't hurt if he read this book. The more he understands about breastfeeding and how important it is for a nursing mother to stay well rested, the more receptive he may become to domestic chores.

Here is a partial list of tasks that Dad can shoulder:

- Drop-off and pickup at daycare

- Laundry

- Shopping

- Cleaning the house

- Fixing meals

- Night feedings (if the baby has been weaned to a bottle)

- Night diaper changes

- Baby-sitting so that you can get out for some fresh air and exercise

- Trips to the pediatrician

II

D-Day

When Delivery Day finally arrives breastfeeding will move abruptly from the conceptual stage to a reality. Let's walk through those first twenty-four hours together and see if we can narrow that often disappointing gap between what you've imagined and the real thing.

THE FIRST FEEDING

When should it happen? As soon as possible. You may have read elsewhere that your baby should be put to breast immediately after the cord is cut and that the sooner the baby suckles, the better it is for both of you. That may be true, but let's be realistic in our definition of *immediately.*

Your birth experience does not end when the cord is cut. There is the smaller but at times uncomfortable matter of delivering the placenta. If you have had an episiotomy and/or torn your perineum, the obstetrician will have to do some repair work. This should not be terribly painful, but you may feel some discomfort. It also means that you will still be in a rather awkward legs-up-and-apart position for a few more minutes. In addition the nurses will need a few minutes to clean up the bed. Having a baby is a messy business.

The bottom line is that for as much as ten or fifteen minutes after delivery you will neither feel like nursing your baby nor be in a comfortable position to do so. Not to worry . . . neither will your baby.

After enduring hours of contractions, he has just been squeezed through an opening no bigger than a softball. Within seconds your baby must remove a cup of fluid from his lungs and perfect a new skill: breathing. He won't feel like nursing for the first ten or fifteen minutes, either. In fact he probably won't have much of an appetite until just about the time you are ready to offer him your breast.

In other words, *immediately* means somewhere between fifteen minutes and half an hour after your delivery. If possible the first nursing should occur in the delivery room. Tell the nurses when you are ready, and don't let them whisk your baby away to the nursery for less critical weighing, measuring, vitamin K shots, antibiotic eye drops, or posed pictures. Breastfeeding should come first.

The first dance. Neither of you has breastfed before, and you shouldn't be surprised if there is considerable fumbling around. Just as when you are dancing, one of you will have to lead and the other will follow. Some newborns eagerly take on the role of leader. Get them within a half an inch of your nipple and they take care of the rest. Natural nursers like this will muckle onto your breast so perfectly the first time that it makes you wonder what lactation consultants are for.

Unfortunately, many babies seem clueless when it comes to nursing for the first time. Instead of cursing Mother Nature for this bit of bad luck, assume the lead. Guide your baby to your nipple and walk him through each stage of attachment. It may go more smoothly if he is naked and your chest and abdomen are completely exposed. This skin-to-skin contact can help stimulate your baby's natural reflexes to nurse. If the room seems chilly, you can ask the nurses to cover both of you with a sheet and light blanket. Avoid using scented soaps, perfumes, and deodorants when you think you are in labor. These unnatural odors may confuse your baby and interfere with some of the cues he will use to identify you as his mother and to find your breasts as a source of nutrition.

MUCKLING ON

The first few days of breastfeeding can be the most frustrating. Getting your baby properly connected to the nipple may initially be very difficult. Don't be distressed if sisters or girlfriends all seem to have stumbled on the correct technique on the first try. You can't count on being among the lucky, so I urge you to assume the worst, hope for the best, and read on.

In coaching you through this first major challenge I'm bound by the limitations of the printed word. This may be a time when you will need the hands-on instruction of a good nurse or lactation consultant. Don't be afraid to ask for help, and certainly don't leave the hospital until you and your baby can consistently make solid contact. There should be a nurse with you for your first attempt. Even if things seem okay to you, the baby may not have taken your nipple properly. If you get things off on the wrong foot and you continue to nurse that way, you may injure your nipples to the point where even the thought of nursing brings tears to your eyes. Breastfeeding education should be high priority for the hospital nursing staff, but if it's not, squawk. Don't be afraid to sound like a nag. Hospitals running on lean staffs to keep themselves financially solvent can lead to seriously overworked obstetrical and nursery nurses. If things aren't going well, ask to see the lactation consultant. Your baby and breastfeeding are important, and you both deserve the appropriate attention. While I may occasionally disagree with lactation consultants when it comes to some things such as scheduling and weaning, they are masters at helping your baby to connect with your nipple. Hopefully you will have at least touched base with a lactation consultant before your delivery. This prenatal contact will come in very handy if you are experiencing a problem with attachment in these first couple of days.

Muckling on is an everyday part of Maine lingo and refers to the process in which a smaller creature firmly attaches its mouth to a larger creature. Piglets muckle onto sows. Ticks muckle onto hounds. Mosquitoes muckle onto your neck. I like the word because, like the word *suckle,* it reminds me of the sound that a nursing baby makes as he is getting started. Terms such as *latched on* and *became attached* just don't quite capture the firm but gentle connection that your baby creates when he is suckling at your breast. I don't mean to offend or be disrespectful in using it, I just think it's the best word to describe an important part of nursing.

Get comfortable. For your baby to successfully muckle on, both of you need to be relaxed and as comfortable as possible. You may be a bit nervous, so let's not make things any more difficult than necessary. Babies are often very sensitive to the emotional landscape. If you are tense, your baby will pick up these vibes and may balk at your breast or become easily frustrated. If your neck and shoulders are tense, you won't be able to relax the rest of your body.

Find a comfortable seated or semireclined position. If your bottom is very sore from the delivery, you may need some help from the nurses or your husband in finding an arrangement that keeps the pressure off your rear end. If you have had a c-section, you probably won't be able to sit up for a few hours, so skip to the section on nursing while lying down (pages 83–84).

Make sure that you have plenty of pillows handy because you will need them to support your arms in the beginning. Eight pounds doesn't sound like a lot, but your arms, neck, and shoulders will quickly fatigue as you cradle your "little" baby for half an hour or more. By supporting your arms on an arrangement of pillows, you can relieve most of the muscle tension that can interfere with guiding your baby into a successful muckling position. For the first day or two you may need an assistant handy to make adjustments in your pillow arrangement. At this stage two hands aren't enough. Don't despair. You will be able to assume a comfortable position without help later on when your arms become accustomed to the weight of your baby.

Get lined up. If your baby is going to get your nipple in his mouth properly, his body and your breast need to be aligned properly. This may seem obvious, but most of us are naturally inclined to cradle a baby in our arms so that we can look him square in the eyes. Unfortunately, that forces the baby to turn his head at an awkward angle to face your nipple. Most babies won't assume this posture, and if they do, they won't do it happily or for very long. Imagine if you were lying down and I offered you a glass with a straw, but made you turn your head 90° to the right to get at it. Trust me, it's uncomfortable!

The proper way to hold your baby is to align him so that his shoulders and hips are facing the vertical plane of your body with his mouth directly in front of your nipple. In the beginning this position may look and even feel a bit awkward. However, it is extremely important to have your baby squarely facing your nipple if he is going to muckle on successfully. You must be comfortable and so must your baby. This position will take the stress off his neck and shoulders and help position your nipple squarely in his mouth. Your assistant may have to help you orient your baby correctly the first few times.

Other positions. If you find that either you or your baby are uncomfortable with the cradle position, or if you just want some variety, there are several other common positions that you can try. One is sometimes referred to as the football position because it reminds some of us of the way a running back carries a football. Support your baby's head on your hand, his legs and feet extended under your arm and out behind you. Remember the goal is to position his mouth to squarely face your nipple. He shouldn't have to turn his neck to reach it.

Another standard position places you and your baby lying on the bed with him facing upward. By leaning on one elbow or resting on a pillow, you can place your breast above his face. You can adjust your position by rolling slightly one way until your nipple is in exactly the perfect position for him to latch on. This arrangement may be more comfortable for both of you, although some women find it creates more tension on their neck and shoulders. Some babies simply don't like it because it is different. One major drawback of this position is that it increases the risk that your baby and/or you may fall asleep while nursing. This could create an unsafe situation in that you might roll onto the baby. Of greater concern is that by allowing your baby to fall asleep while you are nursing, you are likely to become your baby's pacifier, something you want to avoid.

Some mothers find a modification of the cradle position more effective. This position is sometimes referred to as the crossover. It leaves one of your hands free to manipulate your breast while using your other hand (not the crook of your arm) to position your baby's head. With two hands you can more precisely position your baby's mouth over the nipple.

Finding the position that works best for both of you will be a trial-and-error process that lasts several days or weeks. As the baby gets bigger, new positions will evolve as he asserts his likes and dislikes. Some features of your baby's position will probably never change, such as the way he grasps one of your fingers, twists a few strands of your hair, or gently lays his hand against the side of your breast. These little habits offer him a sense of security and would develop even if he were bottle feeding.

Swaddling. Your baby may be one of those feisty little buggers who gets frantic as he tries to muckle on. He may begin flailing his arms and hands in a totally dysfunctional attempt to help the situation. As his hands brush his own cheeks they may trigger a rooting reflex that can turn him away from your nipple, or he may inadvertently push your breast away. Don't get the idea that he is rejecting you. He really does want to nurse, but he is new at it and too excited for his own good. If your baby is a feisty one, swaddle him in a receiving blanket or tuck his hands down underneath your arm. Eventually he will learn how to muckle on without getting excited and you will be able to nurse him without wrapping him up.

Getting his mouth around your nipple. With your body comfortable and your baby's body properly positioned, it is time to guide your nipple into his mouth. This process may be as simple as pulling him closer with your arms, or with your hand supporting the back of his head if you are using the crossover hold. As soon as your nipple touches the skin around his mouth, the rooting reflex will kick in. He will open his mouth and shake his head back and forth until he gets your nipple. He begins to suck and, whamo, he is muckled on! Isn't Mother Nature wonderful?

Unfortunately, not every baby is a very effective rooter from the start and not every mother's nipple makes an easy target. This temporary situation can be frustrating for both parties. Rest assured there are solutions. The answer may be as simple as providing the baby with a little bit of directional help with your (or your assistant's) hand. This must be done carefully but firmly. Don't try to guide your baby by pushing on his cheeks. His irresistible rooting reflex will turn his head toward the direction of the cheek that you have touched. The best maneuver is to grasp the back of his head firmly and then when his mouth is open, quickly and firmly force his head toward your breast with his mouth encircling your nipple. This technique may take some practice. With the help of an experienced assistant you will discover how firm you need to be to achieve a good muckle without further angering your baby. In my experience almost all mothers err on the side of caution. They're not firm enough. If you are holding his head properly, you won't injure your baby and you will be rewarded by finding your nipple well inserted into his mouth.

Troubleshooting. Even if you have gotten everything lined up and managed to get your baby attached, it may not be a proper muckle. For his sucking motion to be effective and comfortable for you, his mouth should be around the areola, as close to its outer margin as possible. Some mothers have very large areolae and it would seem impossible for an infant to completely cover the pigmented area with his little mouth. Sometimes it is! However, most babies can get nearly the entire areola into their mouths. It may take a bit more maneuvering on your part to get your baby into a complete muckle, but it is important to keep trying. I know it's aggravating to take him off your breast if you struggled to get him lined up, but it's worth it to do it. If you allow him to suck for any length of time in a faulty position, you are setting yourself up for a bad bout of sore nipples that may doom your attempts at nursing.

Sometimes the problem stems from your baby's unwillingness to open his mouth wide enough to cover the areola. If you have had a small baby (less than five pounds), the problem may purely be one of size. Unfortunately the only solution may be to use some other temporizing measures such as nipple shields (see page 87), pumping your breasts to stimulate production, and then using bottles for a few weeks until your baby and his mouth have grown. As you can imagine, pumping and bottle feeding for a few weeks is not the most enjoyable way to start your nursing career. Once his mouth is big enough, your baby may have become so attached to the artificial nipple that it can be a struggle to get him to take your breast. This may involve more of a commitment than you want to make, but I urge you to give it the old college try for at least two weeks before you decide that the waiting game isn't one you want to play. This is the kind of problem that can be successfully managed by a good lactation consultant. Don't hesitate to get a second or third opinion if the nursery nurses are telling you to pack it in because your baby's mouth is just too small.

More often the problem is that your baby is just being stubborn about opening his mouth wide enough to muckle on properly. There are several approaches you can take here. The most direct approach is to force open his mouth with your fingers and then insert your nipple (and areola). This is easier said than done. First of all, you have probably already run out of hands. In the beginning there just aren't enough of them to go around, and you certainly aren't going to have one left over to open your baby's mouth. Second, as a new mother, concerned about hurting your baby, you probably won't be forceful enough. Now is another time to call on your assistants. Remembering to avoid touching his cheeks (it triggers rooting), force open your baby's mouth with firm downward pressure on his chin. He won't break, and once he gets the hang of it, feedings won't start with a tussle.

A second technique involves using your finger as a false nipple. It is usually about the same size as your nipple but smaller than your areola and certainly much more maneuverable. By moving your finger around you can trigger your baby to begin sucking. Help him to open his mouth further by inserting a second finger. Now replace your fingers with your nipple. Again this is not easy in the beginning without an experienced set of helping hands. This finger-stimulating technique is also helpful for those babies who seem to have trouble putting their tongue in the correct position. If your baby keeps his tongue on the roof of his mouth where your nipple is supposed to be, your finger can help train him.

Many babies are born with a "tongue tie." This means that the little web of tissue that connects the underside of his tongue to the floor of his mouth extends farther forward than usual. In the old days if the baby was felt to be tongue tied the doctor would snip this bit of tissue with a pair of scissors. The thinking was that if left alone the child would have trouble speaking. Nowadays physicians recognize that a tongue tie is just another example of a normal variation in human anatomy. Most pediatricians will counsel you against having it clipped unless the lactation consultant is absolutely convinced that your baby's nursing problem is the result of his inability to lift his tongue.

Nipple shields. Another technique for dealing with the baby who is having trouble muckling on involves a breast or nipple shield. These gadgets look like a bottle nipple without the bottle or surrounding cap. The original shields were made of rubber just like a traditional bottle nipple. Recently, high-quality examples are made of silicone and are much thinner. The shield is placed over your nipple and then the baby is encouraged to suck on this artificial nipple (with your nipple hidden inside). The nipple shield can be helpful if you have flat nipples or nipples of a shape that your baby has trouble grasping. The main drawback of these shields is that they reduce the efficiency of the milk transfer. From time to time I have seen mothers who mistakenly thought that their baby was getting enough milk because they could see it come through the opening in the shield. The truth is that with a nipple shield, the same sucking effort generally doesn't produce as much milk. That doesn't mean your baby will be undernourished, but keep a close eye on your baby's weight (with the help of the pediatrician), if you are forced to use shields. Another drawback is that sometimes babies get hooked on the shields, and you may have a heckuva time getting your baby to take your own nipple. Eventually you will win this battle of the wills, but it may not be fun.

I suggest persisting with your unshielded nipple until at least the second day. If shields are the solution that works, use them. At least they will allow you to get started. You can deal with the attendant challenges later when your baby is bigger and you are more rested.

Flat or inverted nipples. Two of the more difficult impediments to muckling are flat or inverted nipples. Chapter 9 discusses how to determine before you deliver whether this may be a problem for you and suggests some remedies. Now comes the real test. Can your baby successfully muckle on to your flat nipple? Some babies accept the challenge eagerly and through their own persistence can get their mothers' nipples to stand out.

However, many babies need some help in dealing with a flat or inverted nipple. If this appears to be a problem for you and your baby, one of the solutions is to get out your pump and use it to pull your nipple into an erect position and then present it to your baby. As you can imagine this isn't always easy and is another example of a situation in which one more set of hands would be very helpful. Sometimes even with assistance your nipple may flatten out before you can position the baby for nursing.

Another solution is breast shells. These plastic cups are worn inside your bra and through gentle pressure will force your nipple out so that the baby can grasp on. I suggest that you continue to wear them until your milk supply is firmly established. You may find them an effective remedy for engorgement. When you decide to discontinue their use, don't do it abruptly because this may trigger engorgement. Instead, gradually lengthen the time after each feeding before you place the shells in your bra. When you are at a point that you are wearing them for only fifteen minutes before a feeding, you can stop using them altogether.

Flat or inverted nipples can be a real challenge for both you and your baby. Be patient and persistent. Your lactation consultant may have some positioning tricks.

Working with a poky feeder. If your baby seems lethargic and won't even attempt to nurse, ask the nurses if they think that his behavior is normal. If they seem unsure, ask the pediatrician. Labor is obviously exhausting for you; it can also be stressful for your baby. He may be just sleeping it off. If you miss that little window of time right after delivery when your baby is eager to suck, he may be more sleepy than hungry for the next twenty-four to forty-eight hours. That said, lethargy can also be an important early sign that a baby is sick. Don't be shy about asking the medical staff for their professional assessment.

If the nurses are confident that your baby is just being normally poky, then ask for help gently waking him. Try washing his face, undressing and dressing him, and firmly rubbing his back. The feedings will go much better if he wakes on his own, but sometimes infants need help getting started.

Rooming-in. Ask to keep your baby in the room with you while you are awake. That way you will be right there to take advantage of his short wakeful stretches for another attempt at nursing. If your baby is on the quiet side, the nurses are not likely to notice when he stirs in the nursery and your baby may miss a chance to be fed.

Moistening your nipples. One trick that can help your baby muckle on is to hand express or pump your breast just enough to get some colostrum out. Coat your nipple and areola with this liquid to pique your baby's interest. If you are having difficulty expressing colostrum, you can drizzle some sugar water on your nipple to moisten it.

Taking a break. If both of you are getting frustrated, take a break! If you feel up to it, go for a little walk down the hall, or take a shower, even if you have already taken one. Ask one of the nurses to take your baby for a few minutes. Remind her that you don't want her to give him a bottle. Some nurses may not be experienced in breastfeeding management and yield to their natural inclination to try to calm your baby by stuffing a bottle in his mouth.

Come back to the challenge in a half hour or so. Try another position. If you don't feel like you have a good rapport with the nurse who has been helping you, perhaps another nurse has a trick or two up her sleeve. Don't give up. Maybe the half-hour break wasn't long enough. Things may go a whole lot better if both you and the baby get a few hours of sleep. He is not going to starve or dehydrate in the first few days.

Making sure your baby can breathe easily. If you have large breasts, one of your problems may be that your baby is having trouble breathing because your breast is partially blocking his nostrils. Babies come into the world without much in the way of a nose. Usually this isn't much of a problem, but if they are forced to choose between breathing and eating, they will always choose to breathe. If your baby is nursing, albeit noisily, you don't really have a problem. If he can't seem to breathe and nurse simultaneously, hold your breast back by encircling it with your thumb and forefinger.

This hand hold may be necessary even if your baby isn't having trouble breathing. Some breasts are just too large for a baby to muckle on without some extra help. This technique will also help you guide your nipple (and areola) into his mouth. Be careful to hold well back from the edge of the areola. (You may also use this position to start the milk or colostrum flow just before you put him to your breast.)

Being comfortable. Ask the nurses and your husband for as many pillows as it takes to support your baby so that your arm and shoulder muscles don't fatigue and tense up. This tension can be easily transmitted to your baby and discourage him from nursing.

If the first nursing is delayed. Ideally you'll have a chance to nurse during the first hour after you deliver. Practically speaking, that first opportunity may be unavoidably delayed. You may have developed some unforeseen complications from the delivery. You may be bleeding excessively. Your blood pressure may be too high or too low. A portion of the placenta may not have been expelled. These things happen.

Some of these complications may mean a trip to the operating room. Others may require only that the nurses bother you every fifteen minutes to take your pulse and blood pressure. Your medical problems may make it unsafe for you to nurse your baby at all for the first day or two. Don't worry, we can make it work, but first *you* must be healthy, or breastfeeding can't move forward.

More than likely your baby will be the one who doesn't show up on time for your first date. He has some serious business to tend to immediately after delivery. He must transition from living in a warm fluid-filled environment to breathing the air of the relatively cold delivery room. He may not have begun to breathe on his own and may have required assistance from the obstetrician or pediatrician. This could have meant just a few whiffs of oxygen, or the doctors may have been forced to breathe for him for a few minutes. Fortunately, most babies respond very quickly to our resuscitative efforts and are breathing easily enough to go quickly to their mothers' breasts. However, if your baby hasn't been able to clear enough fluid from his lungs, he may be breathing so fast that it would be unsafe for him to nurse.

Although the first feeding is important, your baby must be healthy or it won't work. If your baby has had a complicated delivery, your pediatrician and the nurses should keep you informed of his progress and explain exactly why nursing must be delayed. Remind them that you want to breastfeed and are eager to start at the first safe opportunity.

Hypothermia. One of the more minor complications that can interfere with your initial breastfeeding is hypothermia. Your baby must rapidly learn to control his body temperatures. This can be a real challenge because he is small and wet and the room temperature may be 25°F cooler than the only home he has ever known. Hypothermia can be a serious problem, particularly for premature infants, but it can usually be prevented or managed by the skin-to-skin nursing I suggested in the last section. Your body heat is a safe and effective way of warming up your baby. Hopefully, the obstetrical nurses know about this technique, but if they want to delay the first nursing because of hypothermia, you may have to "remind" them about it. Ask them to check with your pediatrician if they're resistant to the idea.

What if the first feeding is a bomb? Don't worry! While a good first feeding bodes well for future nursing, an unsuccessful one doesn't have to signal an end to your breastfeeding career. You and/or your baby may be too tired to make a good effort the first time. You may do much better with the subsequent feeding because the nurse on the next shift with that special knack or the lactation consultant has arrived.

Many of the most important and enjoyable activities in your life probably went poorly the first time. Driving a car, dancing, swimming, riding a bicycle, and having sex, just to name a few. Like them, breastfeeding is worth the effort. Don't write it off after the second or third unsuccessful attempt.

How long should the first feeding take? Many first feedings last only three or four minutes because either the baby is tired or most of the first half hour is spent fumbling around. However, if your baby really *muckles* on, should you let him suckle for forty-five minutes? Your advisors' "opinions" may vary widely. In general hospital nurses will advise you to feed with just three to five minutes per side for the first feeding. They will probably also suggest a schedule, adding a few minutes per feeding until you get up to fifteen or twenty minutes per side. The nurses' concerns are based on their observations that lengthy first feedings can lead to sore nipples.

On the other side of the fence are the lactation consultants who feel that there is no such thing as nursing that is too long. I believe there's a middle ground. Think about it this way: If you take a walk in a new pair of shoes that don't fit quite right, you will have blisters after just a few blocks. On the other hand if your new shoes fit nicely, you may be able to walk for a mile or two before you experience any pain. However, you can walk all day comfortably in your old broken-in shoes. The same holds true for breastfeeding. If your baby has attached himself to your nipple properly, you're both comfortable and your nursing coach gives your positioning the thumbs up, you can probably nurse for ten or fifteen minutes.

When it is time to stop nursing, break the suction by edging your finger into your baby's mouth. Failure to do this may injure your nipple. If your baby is still eager to feed, wait fifteen minutes or half an hour, then let him nurse again. Frequent shorter nursings are less likely to cause sore nipples.

If you have a c-section. If you have a c-section, your first feeding will automatically be delayed because it is technically very difficult to breastfeed while on the operating table. Most obstetrical units are aware that you and your baby should get together promptly after the surgery, but it never hurts to remind them that you would like to nurse as soon as possible. If you are presented with a choice of spinal or general anesthesia, be aware that spinal anesthesia usually means a shorter recovery period so you'll be able to breastfeed sooner.

Don't worry if your first feeding is delayed whether by c-section or complications following a vaginal delivery. You still have plenty of time to get the ship launched and underway.

Don't worry about bonding, either. During the 1980s it became fashionable to emphasize the importance of mother-infant bonding. Some experts implied that there was a critical period after birth during which a mother and her newborn had to interact to form a normal parent-child relationship. They warned that if this "bonding" failed to occur during the prescribed window of time, significant maladjustments in childhood behavior could result. Unfortunately, publicity about the importance of bonding created unnecessary worry among new mothers who for medical reasons had to be separated from their babies, even if the separation was a matter of minutes.

It is true that if certain animals are separated from their offspring shortly after birth, these animal mothers will reject their own offspring when they are reintroduced. However, many experienced pediatricians, myself included, were skeptical that this same kind of disordered bonding occurred commonly in humans. Fortunately, the pendulum of professional opinion is swinging back to a more sensible position. Most experts now feel that immediate physical contact is not critical for a normal emotional attachment between a mother and her baby.

You will still form a normal mother-child relationship even if the two of you must be separated for days or even weeks. A premature infant, for instance, or one with a serious medical problem might require treatment in a neonatal intensive care unit. The bottom line is that while breastfeeding may be more difficult to establish if you and your baby are separated for a few days, the separation won't interfere with the formation of a close emotional attachment between the two of you.

12

THE FIRST DAY . . . AND NIGHT

The first feeding is behind you. Maybe it was a bust and you are a bit discouraged, or maybe, on the other hand, you are elated because it was a roaring success. Either way, you're probably keyed up by the experience of having a baby, but it won't be long before exhaustion overtakes you. You probably haven't been sleeping well for a month or more, and you have recently discovered that even a short labor is hard work. Before we allow you to get some much-deserved sleep, there are some important issues to consider.

How often should you nurse your new baby? As often as he wants. For the next week it is safe to assume that if your baby is fussy and wants to suckle, he is hungry and therefore should be put to your breast. Once your milk comes in and your baby is gaining weight consistently, this will change, but for the first two weeks you should be nursing on demand. This is one of the few times when your friends who have chosen to bottle feed will have an advantage, but hang on. It is worth it. This arrangement is temporary, and frequent feedings are an important part of getting your nursing career off to a strong start.

The more often you nurse, the sooner your milk will come in and the sooner your baby will begin gaining weight. Frequent nursing also reduces the possibility that you will become painfully engorged on the third or fourth day. In short, for these first few days you can't nurse too often. You may nurse too long and get sore nipples, particularly if your baby hasn't latched on properly, but the message is worth repeating:

> You can't nurse too often during the first week.

This may mean that your baby nurses three times each hour for a couple of hours and then sleeps for three or four hours (or even more) before he feeds again. This is not a time to think about schedules. As you will learn in the next chapter, routines are very important if you want to have an enjoyable nursing career and hope to continue nursing when you return to work. But for now we want your baby to have free access to your breasts.

Rooming-in? One of the best ways to assure that your baby is fed as often as he should be is to keep him in your room. Almost every study about breastfeeding that I've read includes a recommendation that babies stay in their mother's hospital rooms. This arrangement is associated with a significantly better chance of nursing success.

However, before you decide that your baby is going to room-in, let's make sure that you do it safely. An hour before, your baby was floating around in a pond of amniotic fluid, relying on you to provide him with oxygen and nutrition through the umbilical cord. Within seconds of delivery his body had to make several critical adjustments, among them breathing and regulating his own temperature.

This transition doesn't always go smoothly. Some of the fluid that once filled his lungs may still remain. Valves in some of his major blood vessels that are programmed to convert his circulatory system to an air-breathing mode may not have kicked in with his first few breaths. Abnormalities in his heart or gastrointestinal system, undetected by your prenatal sonograms, may not be evident until after his first few feedings. His first attempts at keeping himself warm may fail, and he may develop hypothermia.

For these and other reasons, your baby should be observed closely during his first twelve hours. Although you may not have a nursing degree, you are to be counted on as one of these observers. You will notice if his color becomes pale or blue. You will hear him choking and notice if he is having trouble breathing . . . if you are awake. That "if" is why many pediatricians are still hesitant to endorse rooming-in for a baby's first twelve hours, even though they realize that close contact is important for successful breastfeeding.

There are several solutions to this dilemma. First, the nurses on the obstetrical floor can organize their duties in what is usually called a mother-baby or couplet plan. This nursing plan assigns one nurse to you and your baby (the two of you are called a couplet) rather than a different nurse to each of you. During the first twelve hours that nurse will be checking on you frequently (at least every hour initially) to make sure that you haven't begun to bleed or develop any other postpartum complications. If your baby is rooming-in, the nurse will also check on the baby, and you will be able to sleep knowing that someone else is keeping watch. Mother-baby, or couplet, nursing is a very popular staffing model and more and more hospitals find that it allows them to safely offer the rooming-in option.

If the obstetrical floor doesn't use couplet nursing, you can ask to keep your baby with you when you are awake, and return the baby to the nursery when you want to get some sleep. You can, and should, make it very clear to the nurses that if your baby wakes, you would like them to bring him in and wake you. Unfortunately, some nurses, eager to protect your precious sleep, will rock or walk your baby so that you can get some more sleep. They may make the even bigger mistake of offering him some formula. Unfortunately these well-meaning efforts can seriously interfere with your initial attempts at breastfeeding.

If you are absolutely exhausted, it may be necessary to keep your baby in the nursery so that you can get a few hours of sleep. You should also ask the nurses to put a sign on your door telling visitors to check in at the nurses' station before knocking. Even welcome visitors can keep you from getting the rest you need to feed your infant as often as he wants.

If your baby does not present any unexpected problems in the first twelve hours, you can feel confident about keeping him in your room when you are sleeping. Remember that in another day or day and a half you will be home. You simply can't watch your baby every minute, and you don't have to. While you're in the hospital, put your baby in the bassinet when you are feeling tired. There are significant dangers associated with sleeping in the same bed with your newborn. Babies have been smothered in bedclothes or by the weight of a sleeping parent. Buzz for the nurse or ask your husband to move the baby into his bassinet if you are still too uncomfortable to do so.

What do you do if your baby is too sleepy to feed? While you must be prepared to nurse your baby as often as he wants, don't be surprised if he's as tired as you are for the first twenty-four to thirty-six hours. While he may have been eager for that first feeding, he may then seem more interested in sleeping for the next day.

Don't become discouraged if the going is a little rough for the first day or so. Ask the nurses and your pediatrician to reassure you that your baby is healthy and that his sleepiness is not a sign of infection. Because a few babies will sleep through feedings they should be getting, try to wake him if he sleeps longer than four hours during the day or longer than six hours at night. Try taking off his clothes, washing his face gently, or rubbing his feet. Ask the nurses for tips on rousing him. Don't be surprised if he isn't eager to feed. Feedings go much better when they are his idea rather than yours.

Should you offer him a pacifier? No! While you will read in Chapter 16 that I think pacifiers can play a role in raising a breast-fed baby, this is a bad time to introduce one. For the first week or two your baby should be suckling at your breasts as often as possible. We don't want to waste any of his sucking energy on a pacifier, and we don't want to confuse him with a choice of nipples.

Once he is gaining weight and you are confident that you can tell when he is sucking just because he is tired, you can try a pacifier. Until that time comes (in a few weeks), don't offer him a pacifier. Ask the nurses to put a note on his bassinet to remind them not to offer him one, either. If they're tempted to give him a pacifier, ask them to bring him to you for a nursing instead. Numerous studies have shown that introducing a pacifier at this early stage discourages good breastfeeding, but some nurses still haven't gotten the message.

Make sure that your baby's hands are uncovered so that he can learn to suck his thumb. This usually takes weeks or even months, but give him an early start. If he seems to be scratching his face, you can ask the nurses to file down his nails carefully with an emery board.

The nurse says your baby's blood sugar is low. Before delivery your baby was getting a steady flow of nutrients through the umbilical cord. His blood sugar was maintained at a level that was similar to yours. Now he is on his own. Some newborns are not very successful at keeping their blood sugar up. This is particularly true if your baby is premature or your blood sugar was elevated during your pregnancy.

Prolonged hypoglycemia can have serious consequences including seizures and brain damage, but fortunately these are rare complications. Still, you can understand why nursery nurses and pediatricians take the situation seriously.

For many years physicians were taught that jitteriness was an important symptom of hypoglycemia. I was trained to order a blood sugar immediately if a newborn seemed at all tremulous. However, after nearly thirty years of practicing pediatrics I have become convinced that most jittery babies do not have low blood sugars. If you can calm a tremulous baby by allowing him to suck on a finger, it is highly unlikely that his blood sugar is low. More reliable symptoms of hypoglycemia are poor color, limp body tone, and low body temperature.

Should the nurse suspect your baby has low blood sugar, she can draw a small sample of blood from his heel and test it in just a few minutes. If the test confirms her suspicion, her instinct may be to offer him some sugar water from a bottle. While sugar water may eventually be necessary, you should offer your baby a chance to nurse first. A mouthful or two of colostrum may be all that he needs.

The nurse can then retest his blood, and if hypoglycemia is still present, then you can offer him some sugar water. This should be administered using a syringe and plastic tube, a spoon, or a medicine cup (see box below). This avoids exposing your baby to a rubber nipple, which may create nipple confusion. Discuss how you'll manage hypoglycemia, should it arise, before delivery with your pediatrician and the nursing staff. Afterward remind the nursing staff that you want to be consulted before your baby is offered a bottle or pacifier. Ask that they put a note on your baby's bassinet about your request.

AVOIDING NIPPLE CONFUSION

When your newborn needs more to drink than your breasts are producing, there are three ways you can give him sugar water (or formula) without using an artificial nipple. My favorite is the syringe-and-catheter technique. The nurse can provide you with a 10-cc disposable plastic syringe and a "feeding tube" that has been cut down to three or four inches. She will show you how to place the tube inside your baby's cheek. With slow, gentle pressure on the plunger you will create a trickle of sugar water. His swallowing reflex will finish the job.

Newborns can also be fed using a teaspoon, medicine cup, or shot glass. Your nurse or lactation consultant can demonstrate how to do this safely, by carefully pouring the liquid slowly onto your baby's tongue. These techniques may take at least four times as long as using a bottle and nipple, but the extra time is a good investment because it prevents nipple confusion.

Occasionally, hypoglycemia is so severe that it must be managed intravenously. Fortunately, most babies have learned to control their own blood sugar by the time they have started their second full day of life.

Nursing can make your tummy ache. The sensation of your baby suckling at your breast sends a potent message to your uterus to contract. These contractions help to return your uterus to its non-pregnant size more rapidly and reduce the risk of hemorrhage. That's the good news. The bad news is that these contractions may create painful cramps. Fortunately, these pains subside over the first week; I have never known a mother to be deterred from nursing because of them.

Attachment woes. You and your baby still may not have learned the secret of attachment. He may be pushing his tongue to the top of his mouth or your nipples may be flattening, making it harder for him to latch on. The frustration can be enough to bring you both to tears. If you don't find answers in the last chapter, then call one or more members of your support team. If the nurses on hand don't seem to be terribly knowledgeable, ask to see the lactation consultant.

While babies can get angry that they aren't able to get anything out of your breasts, most of them are biologically prepared for fasting. While doing research into breastfeeding practices I learned that in some cultures newborns aren't fed colostrum. These cultures believe it's not good for the infant—a direct contradiction to Western medical beliefs. Nevertheless these societies have successfully breastfed their infants for generations—just not for the first few days.

13

Day Two

A new set of worries and problems await you as you begin your second full day of motherhood. You may still be struggling with attachment. And the prospect of going home and leaving behind some of your support group can be unsettling.

> The wide variation in the length of stay after delivery means that it is impossible to predict where you are going to make each of the transitions that breastfeeding requires. I have chosen to describe the most common scenario, in which you would have an uncomplicated vaginal delivery and go home on or just after the second day.

While you're undoubtedly cheered by the thought of being back in your own bed and eating familiar food, you may be struggling with one or more of the following:

Sore nipples. Even if you have been careful about positioning your baby's mouth on your nipple, even if you have been careful to avoid soaps and perfumes, even if you have done some careful preparation, your nipples may be getting sore. In fact they may be *very* sore.

Lucky mothers experience only a bit of pain as the baby latches on, but you may find that you are uncomfortable for the entire time he is sucking. Are there things that you can do? Sure!

- Continue to be careful about attachment and detachment. If not done properly, you can sustain a painful injury. Reread pages 79 to 94 and ask the nurses and/or your lactation consultant to watch and help you make adjustments.

- Keep the nursing periods short, five to seven minutes per side.

- If you can, express some colostrum (or milk) and gently rub it on your nipples after a feeding. Let it air dry. This can be soothing.

- Do not sit around in a milk-damp bra. Whenever possible let the flaps down on your bra and allow your nipples air and light. Sit near a sunny window or a foot or two away from a 75- or 100-watt unshielded light bulb (close enough so that you can feel the warmth). I do *not* mean a sunlamp and I certainly don't recommend direct sunlight.

- Saturate gauze pads with warm saline (saltwater solution) available from the nurses or a local pharmacy, and use as compresses until they cool. Then let your nipples air dry.

- Use lanolin cream (as long as you are not allergic to wool) or a nipple cream recommended by the nurses or your lactation consultant.

- Consider using a nipple shield.

- Consider pumping and feeding your baby your own milk with a syringe and catheter, spoon, or medicine cup. Obviously, if pumping causes more discomfort than nursing, look for another solution.

- If your nipples are extremely sore, red, cracked, and scaling, you may ask your obstetrician to refer you to a dermatologist. Occasionally, extremely sore nipples are a sign of an underlying skin disorder such as psoriasis or seborrhea.

Don't give up. Sore nipples are usually a temporary phenomenon that will improve as your milk comes in. In severe cases some mothers stop nursing and pumping temporarily and offer formula for a day or two to let their nipples heal. As you can imagine, this is far from an ideal situation, particularly this early in the game, but don't despair. Although it may take some time and effort, your milk supply can usually be reestablished. Do not get discouraged and don't allow sore nipples to put an end to nursing. Be patient and ask for help. Good nurses and lactation consultants can teach you how to nurse comfortably.

It's normal for a baby to lose weight. With the exception of babies who have been severely malnourished in the womb, all newborns, regardless of whether they are breast or bottle fed, will lose weight for the first several days. Most of them come into the world with enough fluid and energy stored to tolerate these few days without difficulty.

In a recent Mexico City earthquake a maternity hospital literally collapsed. Several babies survived even though they were not recovered from the rubble for several days after the quake. Remember this when you're nagged by the thought that your baby may not be getting enough to drink from your breasts. If he wants to drink more than you have to offer, he won't be happy about the situation, but remember that his body is prepared to wait. Most of the weight loss is water, which will be replaced quickly when your milk comes in. In fact in most cases pediatricians don't begin to get concerned about a newborn's weight loss until it reaches 10 percent of the child's birth weight. For example, if your baby weighed 10 pounds at birth, your doctor may expect him to lose as much as a pound during his first week.

Ask the nursery nurse to weigh your baby just before you are discharged from the hospital. This will probably not be his lowest weight, but you can use it as a reference point when you go to the pediatrician later in the week. At one week of age your baby probably won't be back up to his birth weight, but he will hopefully be a few ounces above his discharge weight. That's evidence that breastfeeding is working.

Losing too quickly. Although most babies are born with enough body water to keep them going until their mothers' breast milk is established, a few may need a little something extra to tide them over. This should be given in the form of 5 percent glucose water, which the nursery nurses can provide. Plain water will not offer your baby the calories he needs.

If the pediatrician suggests that you give your baby a sugar water supplement until your milk comes in, ask her if you can do it with a syringe and catheter, spoon, or medicine cup (see page 100). This will help avoid nipple confusion. I also recommend that water supplements be given *after* every other feeding and *never instead* of a feeding. You want to preserve enough of your baby's natural thirst and hunger so that he will continue to feed frequently. Stop the supplements as soon as your milk comes in.

Is your baby turning yellow? When the umbilical cord was cut, your baby's body suddenly became responsible for the life-sustaining functions that your body had been taking care of for him. Among them is the recycling of old and injured red blood cells, a task performed in his liver. It may take several days for your baby's liver to get up to speed, and until that time some of the by-products of red blood cell destruction may accumulate in his body. One of these by-products is a yellow pigment called biliruben. In small amounts it is harmless, although it may temporarily impart a yellow cast to his skin and even his eyes. In large amounts biliruben can damage your baby's developing nervous system. Premature and sick infants are more vulnerable to these toxic effects. Jaundice is very common, but jaundice severe enough to cause brain damage is very unusual.

The fact is most of the babies I see in my practice have begun to turn a little yellow by the end of their second day. While first-day jaundice may indicate a blood group incompatibility that could require immediate treatment, in most cases jaundice intensifies for two or three days and then gradually fades away over the next week without treatment.

If your baby has turned a bit yellow on the day you are planning on going home, the pediatrician may order a blood test to measure the biliruben level. If the level is too high, your child (and you) will need to stay in the hospital for an extra day or two while your baby receives phototherapy. This can be done in several ways, but the most common treatment uses a set of specially designed fluorescent lights to break down the biliruben as it circulates through your baby's skin. There are systems designed for home use, but they may not be readily available in your area.

Because dehydration can contribute to jaundice, the nurses may ask you to offer your baby a sugar water supplement after each feeding, which can dramatically decrease the biliruben level. Again, be sure that the water is offered in a way that will avoid the risk of nipple confusion.

Some women secrete a substance in their breast milk that contributes to jaundice, so your pediatrician may ask you to stop nursing temporarily. My feeling is that this is usually bad advice this early in the game. Chances are you are probably producing too little milk at this point to aggravate the jaundice, and we want to avoid interrupting the nursing process just as it is getting started. On the other hand, if your baby's biliruben continues to climb for several days despite usual therapy, it may be necessary to stop nursing *temporarily* (a day or two at most), pump, and give your baby formula to help clarify the diagnosis. However, jaundice is *never* a reason to permanently stop breastfeeding. If you are given this advice, it's time to look for a second opinion.

Jaundice may rarely be associated with a serious infection. If your child begins to turn yellow after you have left the hospital, call your pediatrician. She will ask you a few questions to help her decide whether she can wait until his first office visit to examine him or whether you should bring him in promptly.

Just say no thank you to complimentary formula packs. The manufacture and sale of infant formula is big business. Formula companies know that most breastfed infants will eventually be fed formula, so they want to establish a relationship with you as soon as they can.

You may have already been offered coupons and free cans of formula at your obstetrician's office. The literature that accompanies these gifts is carefully worded to create the impression that the formula manufacturer strongly advocates breastfeeding, and that they are merely interested in helping you keep your child well nourished after you stop nursing.

Although the formula manufacturers do fund and subsidize numerous worthwhile pediatric educational programs, giving new mothers starter packs of formula obviously undermines the breastfeeding process that these companies claim to be supporting. The first week or two of nursing will be the most tiring and the most frightening. There may be times when you are so exhausted or so worried that your baby is starving that you will be tempted to feed him something that you pour out of a can. It will seem so much easier and so much more predictable. You can feel it, touch it, measure it, and see the level in the bottle as your baby sucks down the formula.

Unfortunately, acting out of desperation at two in the morning may herald the end of your nursing career. Your baby may begin to refuse your nipple because the formula came so quickly and easily. It satisfied his hunger and thirst, something your breast hadn't been able to do yet. In your sleep-deprived state you may decide that anything that will give you some rest is an improvement. I have seen this scenario play out hundreds of times.

Instead of reaching for the free can of formula, reach for the telephone and call someone on your support team. One of them will be able to talk you through this frightening and frustrating stage, as I have with many a concerned mother. It would be a shame to abandon your efforts just hours before your milk is coming in. I know of several instances when friends and relatives have climbed out of bed and driven across town to help provide comfort and advice to a new nursing mother.

There is no reason to have a can of formula at home during the first week or two. Your baby won't starve, and its presence will serve only as a temptation to do the wrong thing. There may be a time for formula, but not in the first week. Politely decline the samples if they are offered. In our hospital the pediatricians have requested that formula be excluded from new-mom kits. While coupons may come in handy, just say no thank you to the free formula.

Should you take home a few bottles of sugar water? If you and your baby have made good nipple-to-mouth contact and he seems satisfied with each feeding, there is no reason to take home any liquid supplement. However, if the nurses feel he is looking "dry" (i.e., a little dehydrated) or your baby is unsatisfied after most feedings, it may be a good idea to take home a few bottles of sugar water. While you can make your own, it is much safer to use the sterile and accurately measured 5 percent glucose water that the nurses can give you.

Using a syringe, spoon, or medicine cup (see page 100) to avoid nipple confusion, you can offer him sugar water *after* every other feeding. Your baby can have as much as he wants, but this will generally be less than an ounce. As soon as you suspect that your milk has come in, you should stop the sugar water supplements because they may aggravate engorgement. Most babies do not need sugar water supplements, and those who do require it for only a day. Consult with your pediatrician before supplementing longer than two days.

Be sure to have a breast pump at home. In Chapter 9 I suggested that you put a breast pump on your list of things to buy before you delivered. You may need it to relieve engorgement as early as your first night at home. By the second or third day home you may want to have your husband feed your baby some of your milk in a bottle and give yourself some much-needed rest. In the next chapter you will learn exactly when and how to use your pump. Make sure you already have one when you go home.

Don't go home unless you have had at least one good feeding. As a newborn, I was already gaining weight by the time I went home from the hospital. In those days mothers and their babies customarily spent ten days to two weeks recuperating from the delivery. These days, though, unless you have had a very complicated delivery, you will be going home before your milk has come in fully and probably a few days before your baby has begun to gain weight.

While extended stays are expensive and impractical, it is very important to stay in the hospital until you and your baby have had at least one good feeding. It may not have lasted more than six or seven minutes per side, but you should have felt good suction and been reassured by the nursing staff that your baby was well positioned.

If you have not had at least one good nursing, make sure that you communicate this to both the obstetrician and your baby's pediatrician. They are the people who will write the discharge orders that will release both of you from the hospital. If they don't know that you are having nursing problems, they may send you home prematurely. Even with an excellent support system, you will find it more difficult to get prompt and skilled advice after you have left the hospital.

It's possible your baby hasn't nursed well because he is ill, and you're the first to notice it. No one has been watching your baby as closely as you have. I can think of several newborns who were rescued from serious illness because their mothers refused to go home before they were confident their babies were feeding well.

Your insurance company may have standards that influence how long you can stay in the hospital after delivery, but they are only guidelines. The failure to have a good feeding is a perfectly legitimate reason to stay an extra day or longer. Doctors, hospitals, and even insurance companies can be flexible, but you'll need to speak up to get their attention.

Are your lifelines in place? You've had at least one good feeding. Although you realize that there is still a lot to learn and there are many hurdles to clear, it is time to go home. It may feel scary, but remember that you have established a support team to help you through this transition. Assistance and encouragement should be just a phone call away. Your baby may get hungry and thirsty while he is waiting for your milk to come in, but he isn't going to starve. If the situation gets too frightening, you can always bundle up your baby and return to the security of the hospital for a shot of reassurance. Don't be embarrassed to do it. Sometimes just reminding yourself that the hospital and the nurses will still be there if you need them is enough to keep you going.

Before you go home, make arrangements to have your baby weighed at the pediatrician's office, the hospital's follow-up clinic, or in your own home by a visiting nurse. This first weight check should occur no longer than four days, and preferably two or three days, after you have gone home. At this visit your baby will be weighed to make sure that he isn't losing weight too quickly and the nurse or doctor will examine him to make sure that he is well and neither too jaundiced or dehydrated. This will be your opportunity to ask any questions you might have about breast-feeding and to get face-to-face reassurance that your baby is doing well.

Prior to that visit you will be relying on phone conversations, so make sure that you have the phone numbers you'll need and understand the availability of your support team, which may now include one of the nurses or lactation consultants.

14
THE FIRST NIGHT HOME

You have arrived home. It has taken your husband four trips just to bring in all the gifts and flowers from the car. You are relieved to be in familiar surroundings, but a bit overwhelmed. A new human being, small and vulnerable, is relying on you for his survival.

You are tired, exhausted from labor and delivery and lack of sleep. Unfortunately you can't count on getting long stretches of uninterruped sleep at home, either, but at least you're in your own bed. Although if you have had a c-section or an extensive episiotomy, you may not be able to navigate your way to your upstairs bedroom for a few more days.

Where is the baby going to sleep? For the first week you may feel more comfortable if your baby sleeps in his crib or bassinet in your room. Although in the next chapter I will encourage you to move him into his own room as soon as possible, you will probably find it more convenient to have your newborn sleep near your own bed for now. I don't advise co-sleeping because, like many health professionals, I consider it unsafe and because it can discourage good sleep habits. It is fine to nurse your baby in bed until you feel comfortable nursing in a rocking chair. Hopefully, Dad will be available to ferry his newborn back and forth to his crib for feedings that may be coming as frequently as every hour or two.

Don't even think about schedules. Your baby's feeding pattern in the hospital will probably bear no resemblance to what happens after you get home. He may have fed frequently during the day and slept longer at night, but that will probably be reversed for the next few weeks. On the other hand he may have been a night owl in the hospital and then proceed to send you into a panic by sleeping for six straight hours his first night at home. It is safe to say that there will be no obvious pattern to his feeding at this early stage, so don't look or hope for one.

At this point you should feed him on demand, which may mean he wants to nurse every hour or two, or he may go for two hours, four hours, two hours, and then sleep for six. I suggest that you try to nudge him awake to feed if he is sleeping longer than four hours during the day, or longer than six hours at night. Don't worry if he doesn't wake easily for these feedings. Babies generally feed better if it's their idea.

Try to have him feed on both sides at each feeding. This may mean cutting back to five minutes per side and alternating back and forth several times per feeding until you have figured out how long he is going to nurse on each side. This timing is likely to change once your milk comes in. If you find that no matter how short you make the first side, he won't go to the second, then let him do one side per feeding, but no longer than a half hour per feeding. Just remember to feed him on the other side at the next feeding. You can always train him to take both breasts the following week if he isn't already doing so on his own.

More fumbling. Although you may have thought that you and he had mastered the art of attachment while you were in the hospital, he may have forgotten on the short ride home. It happens all the time. This may make your first night home both frustrating and exhausting. Hopefully, he will have remembered how to get it right by morning, but if he hasn't, call the lactation consultant for a refresher course. If the problem is not corrected quickly, your nipples may become very painful, and your nursing career will be in jeopardy.

15
Days Three, Four, and Five

The next few days will probably be the most difficult for all three of you. Panic, exhaustion, and sore nipples can combine to send many breastfeeding efforts into a tailspin before the first week is over, but with a support group and this book at your side, you'll make it.

The waiting game. In more than twenty-five years of pediatric practice I have met only one woman whose milk came in fully on the first day. She had been leaking large quantities of milk for several weeks before she delivered. Every other mother I have seen has had to endure the uncertainty and frustration of waiting a minimum of two or three days and sometimes as long as two weeks for their breasts to produce enough milk to satisfy their babies.

Waiting for something good to happen can be difficult. If your baby isn't blessed with a patient disposition, waiting for your milk can be unbearable. You both know what he's not getting. You're worried that he might starve. His crying can't be ignored. Exhaustion has drained your patience and disabled your judgment. Don't despair! There are things that you can do to make the wait more bearable, things that won't jeopardize your breastfeeding career.

How long can your baby wait? As I discussed earlier, most babies come into the world well hydrated and with energy stores to keep them going for several days and in some cases a week. However, some babies don't drink enough amniotic fluid during labor and may require more fluid than your breasts can provide in the first few days.

How can you tell if your baby needs a sugar water supplement? Most babies who need extra fluid while they are waiting for your milk to come in won't keep it a secret. They will want to nurse every hour, but unlike the baby who is adequately hydrated they won't be satisfied after ten or fifteen minutes of sucking. If that sounds like your infant, it may be time to offer him some sugar water.

There are a few babies who become dehydrated without much complaint. It may be too content and optimistic by nature, or they simply may not know any better. More important than the cause is for you to learn the signs of dehydration in case you are blessed with one of these babies who is too timid to complain.

SIGNS OF DEHYDRATION

Temperature of 100°F or greater. In the first month, a fever should prompt an *immediate* call to your pediatrician. Although the primary concern should be infection, an elevated temperature may indicate dehydration.

Lethargy. While most thirsty babies will be agitated and eager to suck on anything that gets within a half inch of their mouths, dehydration can eventually cause lethargy. The occasional six-hour interval between two feedings can be normal in the first week or two, but the next feeding should come within three or four hours. If it doesn't, call the pediatrician promptly.

Dry mouth. Your baby's lips may become dry and appear callused. This is normal. After all, they have been working hard against your nipples. However, his tongue and the roof of his mouth should be moist, particularly after a feeding.

Decreased urine output. The new hi-tech disposable diapers are so absorbent that it is sometimes difficult to tell if your baby has urinated. Once your milk has come in, you can expect to find a wet diaper with every feeding, but until then be content with two or three diapers per day.

Brick dust. Like the rest of us your baby has the ability to concentrate his urine when he isn't getting enough to drink. In doing so he saves precious fluid that might have been lost into his diaper. In addition to being darker in color, the urine stain in your baby's diaper may have a pink powdery substance in its center. Because it resembles the material that rubs off of red masonry it is often referred to as *brick dust*. It is actually a sediment of uric acid crystals, which are normally found in urine. These crystals dissolve in toilet bowl water so that we don't notice them in our own urine.

The appearance of brick dust in your baby's diaper does not necessarily mean that he needs a sugar water supplement. It merely indicates that he isn't getting quite as much fluid as he needs. It will disappear as he begins to drink more from your breasts. If he shows no other signs of dehydration, you can disregard the presence of brick dust. However, if it still appears in his diaper after his first week, consult your pediatrician.

How to offer sugar water. I have covered this already, but it is worth repeating because if improperly done, sugar water supplements can discourage breastfeeding.

- Offer the sugar water using a syringe and catheter, spoon, or medicine cup to avoid nipple confusion (see page 100).

- Offer no more than an ounce at a time.

- Always offer it *after* a nursing.

- Offer it after every other feeding to preserve your baby's thirst for your breast.

- Do not offer plain water. Your baby needs an energy source as well as fluid.

- As soon as you suspect your milk is in stop the supplement in order to avoid aggravating engorgement.

- Do not offer formula. There may be a time for it later on, but for now your baby doesn't need it.

THINGS TO DO WHILE YOU ARE WAITING

It may be half a day or it may be three, but regardless of how long it is, the wait will seem to last forever. The arrival of your milk is a biologic process that takes time and is resistant to our attempts at hurrying it along. The more children you have, the sooner it comes in, but that's little comfort to a first-time mother. There are a few simple things you can do while you are waiting that will prepare your body for the challenge of milk production and that *may* speed up the process by half a day or so.

- **Sleep.** This is a good time to learn the trick of napping when your baby sleeps. Parenting and breastfeeding are exhausting. Eight hours of sleep at night, even if it is uninterrupted, will not be sufficient. You need to find a way to grab a few hours here and there, particularly as your body recovers from the exhaustion of childbirth. Don't let fatigue put an end to your nursing career before it begins.

Even if you haven't taken a nap since you were a toddler, try it anyway. Turn down the ringer on the phone, turn off the lights and the television, and lie down on your bed. I bet you'll drift off much faster than you think. Don't worry about missing your baby's cries; your ears are already tuned to their special pitch.

Temporarily shed yourself of all other responsibilities. Let your husband and other members of your support crew worry about shopping and cleaning. In a few weeks you will have regained most of your strength and may not need to nap anymore. However, many mothers find it a habit that, schedules permitting, makes them more cheerful and effective parents. My mother started napping when I was an infant and continued the practice long after my sister and I had given up the practice.

- **Eat.** Many women lose their appetites in the first few weeks after delivery. Although you may rejoice at what appears to be nature's way of helping you get back to your prepregnancy weight, remember that breastfeeding mothers are still eating for two. Don't worry too much about foods that you eat getting into your breast milk (see more in Chapter 19) because you aren't producing much milk. Eat what appeals to you and don't give a thought to dieting.

- **Drink.** Once your milk supply goes into full production you will be losing an additional thirty to forty ounces of fluid from your body each day. That fluid must be replaced and there's only one way to do that: Drink up! Drinking eight ounces of fluid each time you sit down to nurse your baby is enough to do the trick.

It is important to drink a variety of beverages. Milk is a good choice because it is an efficient way of taking in a mixture of nutrients, including protein, carbohydrates and fat. However, if you are allergic to milk, your digestive tract is intolerant of it, or you just don't like the taste, don't force yourself. Talk to your obstetrician and/or a dietitian about other ways of meeting your body's calcium needs.

Although water is important, drinking too much of it can actually decrease your milk production. Our kidneys can excrete more water than we take in if we are drinking too much. In other words excessive water drinking can act like a diuretic. I have worked with several mothers who were having trouble making enough milk until I suggested that they cut back on water and drink more juice and milk. The bottom line is that you should drink a variety of liquids, particularly milk, juice, and water. Stay away from soft drinks and diet drinks. They just don't measure up nutritionally.

- **Pump.** Your body will try to make as much milk as your baby demands. The sensation of rhythmic suction on your nipple sends a message to your brain, which in turn signals your breasts to increase production. Your baby's suckling is the most powerful stimulus. However, if he has been asleep for more than two hours and you are awake, use your pump on both breasts for ten to fifteen minutes. Save anything that you can collect and offer it with a syringe after the next feeding.

Don't be concerned if you don't get anything out. The stimulation alone may still be helpful. Pumping is a skill that not all women possess. If you find that pumping is making your nipples sore, stop.

How will you know when your milk is in? It may not be obvious. While many women notice that their breasts feel firmer and heavier, you may not. In fact some women never see their own milk because they enjoy the fortunate combination of having a baby who doesn't spit up and breasts that don't leak. There are other clues that you are producing milk:

- Your breasts feel larger, firmer, heavier and more tender.

- The liquid dripping from your nipples changes from being thick and yellowish (colostrum) to being thin and watery, with a slight blue tint (breast milk).

- Your baby is more content after feedings and may begin to sleep longer between them.

- You can hear your baby swallowing when he is nursing.

- You see milk in your baby's mouth or when he spits up.

- Your baby may seem uncomfortable and gassy. The first stomachful of milk may give him a belly ache. (Remember, up to this point he has been accustomed to drinking amniotic fluid, which doesn't have much substance and hasn't required digestion.)

- Your baby begins to urinate more and the brick dust disappears.

- Your baby's bowel movements begin to take on a yellow color, eventually resembling a yellow mustard or watery scrambled eggs.

- Your baby begins to gain weight. This is really the bottom line. No matter what you feel and see, if your baby is getting an ample supply of milk, he will begin to gain weight.

Notice that I have not suggested that you count bowel movements or wet diapers. There is such wide variation in the frequency of these functions that you could become needlessly worried if your baby didn't reach or exceeded particular numbers I gave you. If your baby is gaining weight nicely, we don't care how many times he poops or pees on any given day.

Likewise, I urge you to leave the weighing to your pediatrician. Home scales are often inaccurate, and you may be tempted to weigh your baby too often. Because his weight fluctuates throughout the day, you may become unnecessarily concerned when you discover that he has lost an ounce or two. This worry may adversely effect your ability to produce milk. It is seldom necessary to weigh a baby any more often than every other day.

Don't be concerned if you can't hand express or pump much milk from your breasts. I have known hundreds of women whose babies have grown nicely while nursing but who could extract only minute amounts of milk from their breasts with the artificial stimulation of pumping or hand expression.

The let-down myth. You may have heard other women use the term *let-down* to describe the process in which milk is ejected from their breasts. This can be a rather dramatic event in which the milk is sprayed in an ultrafine stream reaching halfway across the room. On the other hand, the flow may start as a heavy and voluminous drip. As a young pediatrician who wasn't equipped with functioning breasts, I had assumed that the let-down process was associated with a sensation similar to that which I experienced when emptying my bladder. However, after listening to hundreds of women, including my wife, describe the feeling, I've learned that many nursing mothers don't feel anything remarkable when milk is released from their breasts. For example, for some women a wet nightgown alerts them to the fact that their breasts are leaking. Other mothers describe a distinct "tingling" feeling when their milk lets down.

Don't assume that just because you don't feel a let-down sensation that nothing is happening. If your baby is having yellow bowel movements and urinating frequently . . . something good is happening.

Engorgement. Up to this point your breasts have been merely ornaments. Now they have to go to work. With that transition comes a certain amount of remodeling. Glands and tissues that have been dormant for about twenty years enlarge. Blood vessels will swell as nutrient-rich blood flows into your breasts providing the raw materials for milk production.

Initially, your body may go a bit overboard in its preparatory efforts and your breasts can become painfully swollen. This is called engorgement and can present a difficult but temporary challenge during this first week. While some of the swelling is due to arrival of milk, a large part of the swelling is distended blood vessels and tissues that will return to a more reasonable size after a few days. Of course your breasts are going to be larger while you are nursing, but don't be fooled by your engorgement experience into buying bras that are too large. Wait a week or so until your breasts have settled down before you purchase new undergarments.

Although engorgement may only last for a few days, it can be frustrating and painful. Your breasts may swell so much that your nipple flattens out and your baby can't latch on. It's a cruel catch-22. If your baby could only latch on, he could extract some milk and relieve some of the swelling. You both know that there is plenty of milk, but he can't get at it. Yes, you can have too much of a good thing.

Here are some things that you can do to prevent and ease engorgement:

- Nurse your baby as often as he wants during the first week. This may keep you a step ahead of the swelling. Stop sugar water supplements (if you're giving them) as soon as you sense any fullness in your breasts.

- Take a warm shower to soften your breasts just before you nurse. This may help your baby latch on.

- Ibuprofen may help. Check with your obstetrician first before taking it.

- Pump your breasts just enough to get your nipple to stand out so that your baby can latch on. (This is one of the reasons I recommended that you go home from the hospital with a pump at the ready.)

- If you are still very uncomfortable, a cold compress or ice wrapped in a towel placed on your breasts may help.

- Wear nursing cups (see page 88) inside your bra. These will help put pressure around your nipples and encourage them to stand out.

While nursing cups can be a great help when you are engorged, don't stop using them abruptly or your breasts may rapidly reengorge. If you feel that you no longer need the cups, wean yourself away from them gradually. Start by waiting fifteen minutes after a nursing before you put them on. Add fifteen more minutes to that waiting period every other feeding until you are wearing them just for a few minutes before the next feeding. It should then be safe to stop.

If you have been wearing nursing cups because you have flat or inverted nipples, you will probably be able to stop using them after your milk has come in. If not, try to wear them only for a few minutes before your baby nurses. A few mothers seem to lose so much milk into the cups that their babies get shortchanged.

THE WAIT IS OVER . . . NOW WHAT?

My milk is in! How often should we be nursing? For the moment the answer continues to be, "As often as your baby wants to feed." He has been fasting for a few days and will probably want to make up for lost time. Your milk may not come in fully at first, but your baby's frequent sucking will stimulate your body to increase its production. On the other hand, your milk may arrive with such force that your baby gets more than he bargains for. With a belly full of milk he may sleep twice as long.

In other words, there is no correct answer to this question. If your baby wants to feed every hour, let it happen. This will help keep you from getting engorged. It will also help stimulate your supply and can give your baby's weight gain a nice jump start.

If your baby seems very satisfied after a feeding and wants to sleep, that's okay, too. However, a few babies will sleep through feedings that they should be getting. Until you are sure you don't have one of these oversleepers, try to wake him four hours after daytime feedings and six hours after nighttime feedings. If he doesn't seem interested after a few gentle pokes, let him sleep. The feedings are much better if it is his idea rather than yours. Waking your baby for feedings is no longer necessary once you've established that he is gaining weight. At that point we can let Mother Nature take over.

If you are becoming painfully engorged because your breasts are filling up before your baby is ready to feed, you can pump . . . but be careful. If you pump too much, your body will interpret it as a demand for more milk and you may aggravate the problem. Pump just enough to ease your discomfort. Eventually supply and demand will balance out as you and your baby fall into sync.

How long should we be nursing? Your baby will probably drain most of your milk during the first five to seven minutes of nursing on each breast, though your baby may feed eagerly for fifteen minutes per side. Nursing for much longer than this may contribute to nipple soreness and will encourage your baby to treat your breast as a pacifier.

It is important for your baby to nurse from both breasts at each feeding because nursing on one side can only discourage the eventual lengthening of feeding intervals. The practice can also be associated with mastitis (breast infection). During these first few days one-sided feedings may be difficult to prevent. Neither you nor your baby knows exactly what to expect. He may find his little belly is full after just eight or nine minutes of sucking on the first breast. Before you both realize what has happened, he falls into a deep sleep.

The solution is to shorten the initial nursing time to five minutes on each side. If he still seems hungry, return to the first breast for a second five minutes, and if he continues to want to suck eagerly, move back for another five minutes on the second side. Continue back and forth until he no longer seems hungry or he has fed fifteen minutes on each breast, whichever comes first. After a few feedings you can begin to lengthen the time on the first breast until you have reached an arrangement in which your baby feeds on both breasts for approximately the same number of minutes.

If your baby is stubborn about nursing on only one breast per feeding, don't fight with him now. If he refuses to take the second breast no matter how much you shorten time on the first side, let him nurse for twenty or thirty minutes. At this stage it is more important that your supply become well established and that he begin to gain weight. You can, and should, try this alternating scheme the following week, when you know he is well above his birth weight.

Some lactation consultants emphasize the difference between fore milk, which is ejected early in the feeding, and hind milk, which is released at the end. They worry that if a baby does not receive enough hind milk at a feeding, he may not grow well. This does not seem to be a common problem in my practice. These experts also feel that hind milk is richer and possibly more difficult to digest for some babies. I have seen several babies who were gassy apparently because their habit of nursing on one side provided them an excess of hind milk. When their mothers coaxed them into nursing on both sides at each feeding, the gassiness resolved.

> To help you remember which side you should start on at the next feeding, place a safety pin on the bra strap of the breast you have finished on.

When should I burp my baby? In the last section I told you not to worry if your baby didn't burp. Chances are he wasn't swallowing enough air and fluid to cause a problem. However, now that your milk is in you will need to pay some attention to burping. In Appendix 1 you will find a detailed discussion of burping techniques. Now let's talk about how often you should be doing it.

Your baby swallows more air at the beginning of a feeding, when he is creating suction and your milk is first ejected into his mouth. If you wait too long to burp him, these large air bubbles will fill his stomach and fool him into thinking he is full, or they will be forced downstream into his small intestine. Once out of his stomach these gas bubbles cannot be burped out and will pass on into his large intestine, where they may give him a stomachache later in the day.

The best plan is to burp your baby halfway through each side and at the end of each side. Don't waste more than three or four minutes per attempt. If you don't get the gas up quickly, persistence may succeed only in making your baby tired and cranky. There is really no harm in putting your baby down without a good burp. It is a process he can do by himself.

If your baby becomes terribly upset by your attempts to take him off of your nipple at the midpoint of each side, don't argue with him. He'll swallow more air only if he starts yelling and screaming. Most babies will pause when they feel a bubble forming in their stomach. Other babies won't stop until they have swallowed so much air that they are too uncomfortable to be burped easily. You'll have to experiment with the best arrangement for your baby. Try earlier rather than later first.

Why does my milk look so watery? While breastmilk is clearly the best first food for your baby, it certainly doesn't look the part. You may have been expecting to see something rich and creamy, but your breastmilk could pass for dirty dishwater. It is thin and watery and makes skim milk look robust. Don't be disappointed; that's what breast milk is supposed to look like.

An ounce of formula contains twenty calories and so does an ounce of your breast milk. To approximate the nutritional content of breast milk, the formula company scientists have been forced to thicken their product. This means your breast milk has more water, which promotes kidney function and digestibility and prevents constipation. While your breast milk may not win any beauty contests, it is still the best food for your newborn.

More about sore nipples. You may have escaped sore nipples while you were in the hospital, but the frequent feedings of the last few days may have taken their toll. Try rubbing a little breast milk on your nipples as a soothing lotion.

Your nipples may crack and bleed, although you may not notice this until your baby spits up some blood-streaked milk. Don't panic; this is a very common occurrence. If you can find a crack in your nipple that is leaking blood and your baby seems fine, you can wait until morning to call the pediatrician for reassurance.

On the other hand, if there is more than just a little streaking in the spit-up and you can't find a crack or your baby seems weak or pale, you should call the doctor immediately. Ninety-nine percent of the time the blood your baby has vomited is your own, and your baby is in no danger. The blood may upset his stomach a bit, but it is usually not a reason to stop breastfeeding.

If your nipples are so sore than you cannot bear to nurse, take a break for several feedings and ask your baby to limp along with some sugar water. He may not be happy, but he'll forgive you once he starts nursing again. Of course if the pain continues to be intolerable after this brief respite, talk to your lactation consultant and/or your obstetrician. If they suggest a longer rest period, talk to your pediatrician about giving formula (by syringe, spoon, or medicine cup if possible) for a day or two while you are healing. If you can pump without further damaging your nipples, do so. This will encourage your body to produce milk.

When you are ready to try nursing again you may have to supplement with formula after every other feeding while you rebuild your supply. This can take as long as a week. Keep in close contact with your pediatrician so that she can help you decide when it is time to stop the supplements.

Your milk is in but you are exhausted. While some babies start sleeping longer once their mothers begin producing milk, your baby may be so eager to make up for lost time that he wants to feed every hour or two around the clock. Obviously this can be exhausting. In your sleep-deprived state you may become cranky, irrational, tearful, and easily discouraged. On top of that, fatigue can interfere with your body's efforts to make milk.

- At the beginning of this chapter I urged you to nurse your baby as often as he wishes, but sometimes you simply can't keep pace; nor could anyone else, for that matter. If you reach this state of exhaustion, offer your baby a formula supplement at night so that you can get some sleep.

Don't be a martyr. There are ways to get some life-sustaining sleep and not only preserve but also boost your nursing. Here's how.

1. If you can pump some milk, do so after as many *daytime* feedings as you can. Store it in two-ounce portions in the freezer.
2. If you can't pump anything, send your husband out for some formula.
3. The first time that your baby wakes after 11 P.M. have your husband get up and feed the baby no more than two ounces of the stored breast milk (or formula), preferably

using a syringe and catheter, spoon, or medicine cup. However, at this point a bottle probably won't cause nipple confusion.

4. Ask your husband to feed him somewhere other than your bedroom so that you can take advantage of this opportunity to sleep. The baby's bedroom would be the best choice.

5. This supplemental feeding can be repeated every other feeding until daybreak, when hopefully you will be more rested.

You could re-create this scenario the next night, but if it is repeated too often you may discourage your milk production. Remember, this is a *temporary* remedy for a serious case of fatigue that threatens to end your nursing career. For the scheme to work you need to grab every opportunity during the day to nap and take advantage of the extra few hours of night sleep that your husband's participation makes possible. If you find that you can't sleep as your husband feeds the baby, you might as well nurse and try to get some rest at another time.

THE F-WORD

Breastfeeding advocates and consultants might cringe at the idea of offering a formula supplement, particularly this early in the game. To them *formula* is the "F-word." However, as I told you earlier, for me the "F-word" is *fatigue*. I agree that when given in the wrong setting formula can set nursing into a tailspin from which it often doesn't recover. But I have seen many more breastfeeding experiences terminated prematurely by fatigue. If you follow the guidelines that I have outlined and remain committed to nursing, you will find that an ounce or two of formula once or twice on one of those horrible nights will keep you on track with breastfeeding.

Unless a strong milk allergy runs in the family, any of the usual formulas should be fine. Otherwise, choose a soy formula.

Remember you are feeding him very small amounts. Formula isn't poison. If an ounce or two of it allows you to regain enough strength to continue a nursing career that will last for several months, the benefits certainly outweigh any minimal risks.

You may be asking yourself how I can make such an about-face after I have adamantly argued for you to leave the complimentary formula pack at the hospital. The decision to offer supplement in the first day or two after your milk has come in is one that should not be taken lightly. It is really a last resort to consider only after you have been unsuccessful in pumping any breastmilk. If it means that your husband has to run out to the convenience store in the middle of the night, that's okay. He may find that by the time he gets home the situation has resolved itself.

In later chapters I will discuss how to introduce formula when you leave the baby with a sitter or return to work. The issues that must be considered in those situations are much different than the fatigue-induced crisis that I have just described.

16

IS MY BABY GAINING WEIGHT?

The one-week weight check. Your baby's first weigh-in is such an important component of a successful breastfeeding experience that I urge you to schedule the appointment before you leave the hospital. Some hospitals offer at least one free follow-up visit as part of their marketing strategy to draw expectant mothers to their doors. In other communities, outreach nurses may come to your home to see how you and your baby are doing. Although there are advantages to both of these arrangements, I have found that the first weight check is most productive if performed by your pediatrician. Her office will be your child's medical home for the next eighteen years, so it's a good idea to get acquainted with the office staff and become accustomed to calling them when you have questions about your baby's health.

Ideally your visit should be three or four days after you have gone home from the hospital, certainly no longer than one week after your baby's birth. If you wait until your baby is two weeks old, he may have lost enough weight to jeopardize his health, and you and he may have developed counterproductive habits that are difficult to break. On the other hand, it's never too early to visit the pediatrician if you are concerned that the nursing is going poorly or if your baby is ill.

Allow yourself extra time to mobilize your new family and get to the doctor's office. It will take at least twice as long to get ready for the visit as you might think. You are new at dressing a baby, and your newborn is likely to have a massive bowel movement just before you leave the house. In fact, if it is wintertime and you live in the northern half of the country, you should count on dressing to take at least an hour. You will become more efficient as the months roll on, but it can be a steep learning curve in the beginning.

Don't trust your memory. Make a list! You won't have forgotten your baby's birth weight, and I hope that you still remember her weight on the day she left the hospital (you can always call the nursery if you don't). You will probably have at least twelve questions that you will want to ask the doctor, but on the ride to the office half of them are likely to disappear into the sleep-deprived fog that envelops the brain of most new mothers. The solution is to write down your questions as they occur to you.

I may not be able to transform you into a compulsive list-maker like me, but I know from experience that your trips to the pediatrician will be much more productive if you arrive with questions on paper. Some less experienced physicians may be irritated or even intimidated by a parent with a list, but I find that it actually streamlines the office visit and greatly increases its value. Don't be afraid to walk in with a list of twenty questions. If you honestly don't have any questions, write down the ones your mother or your mother-in-law has been asking. Let the pediatrician help silence their badgering.

Ask to be put in an exam room as soon as you arrive. Despite what your intuition might tell you, pediatricians' waiting rooms have not been shown to substantially contribute to the spread of disease. However, for very new babies, even a cold may be a devastating event. The sooner you can get into the relative isolation of an examining room, the better. More important, you may want to feed and/or change your baby in private.

Your pediatrician's office staff should be sensitive to the needs and concerns of brand new parents and hustle you into an exam room as soon as you arrive. Don't be afraid to ask if they don't.

A shot of confidence. The nurse steps back from the scale and says, "Congratulations, your baby is gaining weight!" That's the news you have been waiting for. You were thrilled by the sight of the first yellow poop two nights before, and the milk stains on the front of your nightgown have been reassuring, but this is solid evidence that you are able to nourish your baby. The eleven other questions you have accumulated no longer seem important. Good thing you wrote them down.

There will still be hurdles to clear, but now you can relax and really begin to enjoy motherhood. Your baby won't be receiving her first injection for another three weeks, but you have just been given a shot of confidence that should protect you from worry for at least another month.

Nothing gained . . . nothing lost. On the other hand, the one-week weight check may not provide you with the boost you had been hoping for. Your baby's weight may still be the same or slightly below his last measurement in the hospital. Don't get discouraged. About half of the babies (including the bottle-fed ones) I see at one week of age haven't climbed back above their discharge weight. Remember, your baby was still losing weight for the first couple of days that he was at home. We expected him to lose nearly 10 percent of his body weight. He may have begun to gain weight yesterday, just not enough for us to notice yet.

If you have been leaking and your baby is content and having yellow bowel movements, we know that your milk is in. We just need to wait another couple of days and weigh him again to prove that he's growing. The pediatrician has examined him to reassure you that he is healthy and not dehydrated. I know it is disappointing to discover that he hasn't gained yet, but try not to worry until his next visit in a few (two or three) days. Continue to nurse as often as he wants to feed and you will be rewarded with a number that confirms what we already suspect . . . the breastfeeding is working and your baby is beginning to grow.

What happens if your baby is still losing weight? If your baby is losing weight briskly at the one-week check or has failed to gain weight at the second weight check, it is time to explore the causes and consider some changes. Let's look at the most likely causes:

- He may not be latching on properly. The pediatrician may ask to watch you nurse and/or she may have you see the lactation consultant. The solution may be as simple as changing positions or training your baby to suck using your finger.

- Your baby may be sick. Ask the pediatrician if she thinks this is a possibility. She will examine your baby and may do one or two lab tests to rule out the possibility of infection.

- You may be ill. How have you been feeling? Have you been feverish? Overtired? Or suffering any unusual discomfort? Go to your obstetrician for a checkup in the next day or two. Don't let them put you off for a week. You want this breastfeeding problem solved now!

- Have you been eating and drinking enough? It is not unusual for your appetite to dip after delivery. However, it may be a sign that you are ill. Don't worry too much about eating a "healthy" diet at this point. Focus on your favorites for the next week or two, and remember to drink a variety of fluids, at least eight ounces with each nursing.

- Maybe we just need to be patient. Some women take as long as two or three weeks to completely establish an adequate milk supply. A complicated delivery may have set you back a week or so. It is too early to say that you won't be able to keep up with your baby's nutritional needs. Of course not every woman can produce enough milk to keep her baby growing. It does happen, but far less often than people think. Most mothers who are told that they have an "inadequate milk supply" have the potential to make enough milk but lack adequate advice and support. It may take as long as a month to determine that your baby may routinely require a small supplement to grow. For now let's maintain our positive attitude and be patient. Remember, your baby has been examined and will continue to be weighed frequently. That is your safety net.

Is it time to consider a formula supplement? This is an issue to discuss with the pediatrician. If you have selected a pediatrician who is knowledgeable and supportive of breastfeeding, she will be very hesitant to suggest a formula supplement at this point because she knows that even if done carefully, it can interfere with nursing. However, she will look carefully for evidence that your baby needs more nourishment and will tell you when it is no longer safe to simply wait.

On the other hand, if your pediatrician is not terribly experienced with managing nursing problems, she may encourage you to supplement before it is necessary. If you suspect that is the case, don't hesitate to ask for a second opinion.

We can assume that if your baby has not begun to gain weight he will be hungry. We might expect him to be fussy, discontented after feedings, and eager to eat as often as every hour. It isn't cruel to allow your baby to be hungry for a few more days as long as he is healthy. His hunger will motivate him to nurse more often and stimulate your body to produce more milk.

Some babies never complain even when they are getting seriously shortchanged. They may become more apathetic with the fewer calories that they consume. Therefore it is not safe to assume that if your baby isn't complaining he is getting enough to eat. The pediatrician will be looking for other evidence that it is time to offer a formula supplement. Is the baby having trouble keeping his temperature stable? Is his jaundice worsening? Is he making enough urine? Does he look dehydrated? When the pediatrician feels that it is an unhealthy situation, she will suggest a formula supplement.

HOW TO SUPPLEMENT

- Choose a low-iron cow's-milk–based formula (unless there is a strong family history of cow's-milk allergy, in which case choose a soy-based formula).

- Ready-to-feed formula that requires no preparation is the best choice for now. It is more expensive, but we want to save you as much time and energy as possible at this stage. If a long-term supplement is required, then a concentrate or dry-powder product makes more economic sense.

- Offer the formula using a syringe and catheter, spoon, or medicine cup to avoid nipple confusion.

- Offer the formula no more frequently than after every other feeding.

- Unless you are battling severe exhaustion (see The F-Word, page 127), every supplement should be preceded by a nursing attempt.

- For now, offer no more than two ounces of formula at a time. This will help preserve your baby's hunger and keep him nursing frequently. If the supplement becomes routine, then this limit will be removed.

- The formula portion of the feeding should take no more than twenty minutes.

- If your baby sleeps longer than two hours after a daytime feeding, pump your breasts to stimulate milk production.

EXPECT A CHANGE

> When your baby is drinking formula his bowel movements will probably be darker and firmer. If he is getting a soy-based formula, they may even be grayish green in color.

It's all about attitude. If your pediatrician has suggested a supplement, it is tempting to view this as defeat and the beginning of the end of your nursing career. Please don't! You and your baby have been at this only a week or two at most, and there is plenty of time for you both to learn how to do it better.

There are a host of reasons why your milk supply may not be sufficient. You may have an undiagnosed infection; once identified and treated, you'll more than likely start to produce more milk. You may be more fatigued than you realize; a few days down the road, you may feel more like your old self and your breast-feeding may be more effective. You may be tense and anxious about this new responsibility; the safety net of a formula supplement may relax you and you may find your breasts begin to make more milk. I have seen that happen scores of times. Your baby may be a slow learner or still recovering from delivery; once he gets stronger and learns to suck more effectively, your body will respond to his demand.

In other words, look at this formula supplement as a temporary solution to a temporary problem. It is not the beginning of the end, it is merely a strategy to buy us some time to allow you and your baby to rest up and learn.

17

WEEK TWO: WINNING THE BATTLE AGAINST FATIGUE

You are relieved that your baby has begun to gain weight. Life is still chaotic, but you are no longer as worried as you were a few days ago. Though there are still challenges ahead, we can begin to tinker just a little with your baby's schedule to help you get some much-needed rest.

COPING WITH THE DAY/NIGHT FLIP-FLOP

Almost every newborn, whether breastfed or bottle-fed, goes through a period shortly after birth when he gets his days and nights mixed up. That is, your baby would rather sleep during the day and stay awake at night.

Many parents compound the problem by altering their own schedules to match their baby's alert nocturnal state. They may start watching late-night television or leave the light on to read. Even worse, they may stay up and do the laundry or clean the house at one in the morning, figuring that they might as well be productive because if they're going to be up with the baby, anyway. . . . Unfortunately, the sleep debt incurred in the wee hours of the morning is never repaid, because, although a baby naps during the daytime, his parents do not.

The day/night flip-flop will eventually resolve after a few weeks, more quickly if you follow these simple strategies:

Lights out from 7–7. From about seven o'clock at night until seven o'clock in the morning, leave your baby in a darkened bedroom lit by only a small knee-high nightlight. Perform all of your baby care—including feeding and diaper changes—in this darkened environment. Your eyes will adjust to the dim light. Resist the temptation to play or chitchat with him after these nocturnal feedings. Burp him and return him to his crib or bassinet and allow him to fall asleep on his own.

From seven in the morning until seven in the evening, your baby should sleep in this same darkened environment. Opaque, well-fitting shades can help achieve the correct atmosphere. For daytime feedings bring your baby out into the family or living room. After these nursings you can play with him and engage him in conversation, if he is interested. After no more than fifteen or twenty minutes of activity (or sooner if he seems tired), return him to the darkened bedroom for sleep.

This manipulation of his exposure to activity and light will help him "understand" that daytime is a more stimulating and interesting time and that night is better suited for sleeping. Do not interpret my suggestion to mean that you should be keeping your baby up during the day to tire him out so that he will sleep better. Experienced and successful parents will tell you that strategy doesn't work. In fact the overtired infant will usually sleep less well and for shorter intervals.

Notice that I have suggested choosing seven in the evening as your baby's bedtime, not nine or ten or eleven. He is a little child and should have a bedtime several hours before yours. You need that personal time after he has gone down for yourselves and your marriage. Initially, the evenings will be filled with feedings and diaper changes, but in a few weeks you'll be changing and feeding him less often, and you will have that time for yourself. If you don't build that early bedtime into the program now, it will be difficult to introduce it later on, after bad sleep habits have been formed.

Don't stay up because you know your baby will be awake. The real problem with the day/night flip-flop is that parents adjust their lives to become more nocturnal. Resist the temptation to stay up and putter around. Go to bed at a decent hour. There's nothing wrong with going to bed as early as nine while you are still trying to recover from labor and delivery. Grab those extra few hours of sleep when you can. You will be a healthier and happier parent if you keep your sleep debt to a minimum.

Nap when your baby naps. I recommended this strategy earlier, but it bears repeating. Take advantage of the rest time when your baby is sleeping. Turn off the phone, get comfortable, and take a power nap. Don't worry, your ears are tuned to his noises. You will wake when he is ready to feed again.

Move your baby into his own bedroom. It will become very clear as you read on that I don't think bed sharing is an effective child-rearing strategy for most families. If you are going to be a well-rested parent and maintain the stamina that breastfeeding requires, your baby should learn to sleep independently sooner rather than later. The first step in the process is moving him into his own room.

Babies are noisy sleepers and your infant's snorts, rustles, and irregularities of his normal breathing pattern are likely to interfere with your sleep. In addition, your presence in the room can create a distraction that may make it hard for him to put himself to sleep. Of course it's more convenient for night feeding to position his cradle at the foot of your bed, but resist the urge to do so. Instead put him in his own room and enlist Dad to do the footwork at night to bring the baby to you for a nursing. The advantages of having your baby sleeping in a separate room far outweigh the disadvantages.

Don't worry about hearing him if he needs you. Even when you are asleep, your maternal auditory system is tuned to your baby's frequency. I don't generally recommend infant monitors because most young families live in small homes in which sounds travel easily. However, if your bedrooms are on separate floors, you may want to consider using one.

MASTITIS (BREAST INFECTIONS)

With your breasts working at full capacity to manufacture milk for your baby, bacteria can enter the system, usually through a crack in your nipple that may be too small to see or feel. Although your body has a variety of defenses against these germs, infection can still occur when milk flow is slow or interrupted.

You may occasionally notice unusually firm areas in your breasts. These represent portions of your mammary duct system that have not drained fully. This is not unusual, but unfortunately, these areas are more likely to become infected because the normal cleansing flow of milk is impaired. Many women will notice that one particular region of their breast is more likely to plug or harden up. Sometimes this is the result of previous breast surgery, but most of the time it goes unexplained.

Simple ductile plugging is easily managed by making sure that particular breast is emptied well by nursing or pumping. If an infection occurs, the firm area will also become very tender and may even appear red. You may have chills and fever and feel ill. In fact, some women go to the doctor suspecting they have the "flu" because they feel so sick that they don't notice their breast discomfort.

The treatment for mastitis usually requires antibiotics. Your obstetrician will know which medicines are safe if you are breastfeeding. However, if you are being treated by another physician who is not accustomed to working with nursing mothers, make sure that she has checked that the medication is compatible with breastfeeding. You can also take acetaminophen or ibuprofen for the pain and fever.

Apply warm moist heat to your breast and make sure that the milk continues to flow on a regular basis by nursing your baby or pumping every couple of hours. Mastitis is almost never a reason to stop nursing, even temporarily. In fact your child can help resolve the problem by emptying your breasts.

To prevent mastitis, make sure that your bras and breast pumps are clean and dry. Your breasts should be kept clean, but remember to avoid soap. Washing with warm water and air drying is the best approach. Avoid long intervals between feedings or pumping to discourage ductile plugging. Eventually we want your baby to sleep longer intervals, but if you are a woman prone to mastitis, this could present a dilemma. On the one hand, more frequent feedings will keep your breasts flowing more freely, but on the other hand, the schedule can be exhausting. At least one survey of mothers who had suffered with mastitis reports that "fatigue and stress" were more important factors than duct plugging or schedule changes in the development of the condition. This is just one more reason that we have built your Maternity Leave Breastfeeding Plan around fatigue prevention.

Hopefully, you will never get mastitis, or at worst suffer only a single episode. However, there are some women who despite proper technique, hygiene, attention to scheduling, and fatigue prevention have repeated breast infections. The situation can become so uncomfortable and frustrating that they stop nursing. If you are tempted to give up breastfeeding because of recurring episodes of mastitis, don't be afraid to ask for a second opinion about treatment options from another obstetrician or lactation consultant.

WHAT CAN I EAT?

You can probably eat just about anything you would like. Most of the stories you have heard about the relationship between what a nursing mother eats and the behavior of her baby are not worth repeating. In my experience, the majority of breastfeeding babies don't seem to care one way or the other what their mothers have eaten.

There has been very little scientific research on the subject, but what little there is suggests that some infants *may* become gassy and colicky if their mothers eat cruciferous vegetables, which include cabbage, Brussels sprouts, cauliflower, and broccoli.

Other food stuffs which have been implicated are onions, chocolate, and cow's milk. However, before you begin to eliminate these foods from your diet, please read the section in which I discuss the causes of colic (see page 145). What you eat is probably one of the least important factors in the development of your baby's symptoms. I urge you to consider other remedies such as burping and sleep management before you make any severe restrictions in your diet.

For many women, avoiding cruciferous vegetables and chocolate is a minor adjustment, but eliminating cow's milk is much more difficult. Before you decide that you have discovered an offending foodstuff, reintroduce the suspect food again several times separated by a week or more and observe your child for symptoms of intolerance such as spitting up or discomfort. There are so many other compounding factors that it's difficult to be sure what role your diet is playing in your baby's behavior.

Listen politely to the advice of other breastfeeding mothers about your diet, but take what they say with a grain of salt. You and your baby are a unique pair. Just because another mother has experienced difficulty with a certain foodstuff doesn't mean that you will have the same problem. I will remind you again, most mothers can eat a broad and healthy diet without it bothering their baby. In fact there is some preliminary evidence that breast-fed babies whose mothers ate a variety of foods were less likely to be picky eaters as toddlers.

If you notice that your baby is consistently uncomfortable when you drink cow's milk, be sure you discuss your diet and the need for calcium supplements with your doctor before you undertake a long (more than a month) trial of a milk-free diet. There is no need to worry about your calcium intake while you are doing an experiment that takes only a week or two.

18

WEEK THREE: "I WILL NOT BECOME A PACIFIER . . ."

If there's one message I want readers to hear loud and clear, it's that you can nurse your baby without becoming his pacifier. Now that your baby is gaining weight and you are becoming more confident that you can tell the difference between his hungry cry and his sleepy cry, it's time to take a few simple steps to make sure that your breasts don't become part of your baby's bedtime ritual.

You might be wondering what the big deal is. What's wrong with nursing a baby to sleep? At the moment it may seem natural. You feed him for ten or fifteen minutes on the first side. You switch to the other side, and after nine or ten minutes he falls asleep and you put him in his bassinet. He's contented and the silence is heavenly. Unfortunately, with each nursing your baby is forging a stronger association between breastfeeding and falling asleep. Within a very short time (in fact it may have happened already), he will believe that he can't fall asleep without your nipple in his mouth.

If you intend to go back to work or if you hope to have any time for yourself, if you want to be able to go jogging with a friend or out to dinner with your husband, you will find it difficult, if not impossible, to do so if you become a pacifier. You will have to be available twenty-four hours a day whenever your baby needs to fall asleep.

At present each time your baby wakes he's more than likely hungry, and of course he should be fed. However, in just a few days or weeks his immature sleep patterns will be causing him to wake even when he's not hungry. Ironically these "arousals" are more likely to occur if your baby is overtired. I know that doesn't make much sense, but unfortunately these wakings occur quite frequently and have confused and frustrated hundreds of thousands of parents.

If your baby has developed an association between suckling at your breast and falling asleep, he will want to nurse whenever he has one of these arousals even though he isn't hungry. Imagine how tired you will become if your baby is having four or five arousals each night in addition to his usual hungry wakings.

Fortunately, thousands of mothers have avoided this trap, because they have learned how to successfully breastfeed their babies without nursing them to sleep. What these women have done is to coax their babies into learning sleep independence and in doing so have become well-rested and happy parents.

Not everyone believes that children can or should learn to put themselves to sleep. The family bed/cosleeping advocates might argue that my suggestions are cruel and unnatural. Unfortunately, there isn't enough data to favor one method of child-rearing over another. I am willing to admit that some well-adjusted children have come out of family beds. However, in more than twenty-five years of watching thousands of parents raise their children, I have found that for most families, fostering sleep independence works better in our society. The children who have learned to put themselves to sleep aren't any more insecure than cosleeping children, but their parents are certainly better rested.

Some advocates of independent sleeping don't suggest tinkering with babies' sleep patterns until they are four or five months old. However, by the time your infant is six months old, "bad" associations have become firmly entrenched and you are so exhausted that some days you question your decision to become a parent.

Now, before your child is a month old, is the time to avoid those associations that can make you into a human pacifier and leave you feeling trapped by breastfeeding. The first step is simple. Shorten each feeding by a minute or two until your baby is finishing most of his feedings awake. The soporific quality of warm breast milk is so strong at this age that it is unreasonable to expect that your three-week-old baby will finish every feeding awake. It just won't happen, particularly at night. Sometimes he will go from vigorous sucking to being dead asleep in the bat of an eye. Often burping will serve as a gentle wake-up call, but don't count on this occurring and certainly *do not* try to shake your sleeping baby. Merely shorten the next feeding by a minute or two.

The second step is to put your baby in his bassinet or crib while he is awake. If it is daytime (see the discussion of 7–7 on page 137), you may want to play and chat with him for a while (no more than fifteen or twenty minutes at this age), but don't allow him to become too jazzed up or overtired. Overstimulation can make it more difficult for him to fall asleep and is likely to trigger an arousal or nonhungry waking in the next hour or two.

If he begins to cry after you have put him down, resist the temptation to pick him up immediately. This is difficult, I know. If you can wait two or three minutes, you are doing great. Do the minimum to quiet him. Start by rubbing his chest or belly, and comfort him with your words. Pick him up as a last resort. You can walk him around the room, but don't turn on the light. Don't take him out of his bedroom and certainly don't nurse him. Your goal is to stop the crying and then return him to his crib awake so that he can learn to put himself to sleep. If he begins to cry again, leave the room and try to wait a minute or two longer than you did the first time and then repeat the process again (and again!) until he eventually falls asleep in his crib. At this age (less than four weeks old) don't push the process longer than an hour and a half past the previous feeding. You don't want to hold out on a hungry baby. Offer him the chance to nurse. If he falls asleep after just a few sucks, he wasn't hungry and the next time you can wait a bit longer. It may take a week or two for your baby to learn to put himself to sleep without nursing, so don't give up. The important thing to remember is that you don't want to become his pacifier. Particularly if you are going back to work, you can't allow yourself to become part of his falling-asleep ritual.

> For a more thorough discussion of sleep management, I hope you'll read one of my other books, *Is My Child Overtired?* (Simon & Schuster, 2000).

Colic. If your baby is starting to have fussy spells that don't seem to be caused by hunger, you may begin to wonder if you are dealing with colic. Friends and relatives will offer a variety of cures, but be careful. Colic is not a disease for which there is a cure. It describes the behavior of an infant with episodic fussiness which may be due to any one of a hundred explanations. Your first call should be to the pediatrician. She will weigh your baby to make sure that his crankiness isn't due to hunger, but she will also examine him and may do a few laboratory tests to rule out any medical causes.

Sleep deprivation. With these factors eliminated, the most likely causes of his colicky behavior are fatigue and/or swallowed air ("gas"). It may be difficult to accept that notion that your baby's screaming is a result of being overtired. He sounds as though he is in pain, and he may be. Sleep deprivation can trigger migraine headaches in older children, and it is not unreasonable to assume that your infant may be suffering some kind of pain due to lack of sleep. Unfortunately, he can't tell us where it hurts.

You may be surprised to learn that your three- or four-week-old should be sleeping somewhere between fourteen and sixteen hours each day. If he is falling short of that, you can begin to look for places to extend his sleep time. Are you allowing the feedings (including burping) to drag on for an hour or more? By now you should have improved your efficiency so that you can complete the process in forty-five minutes, including a diaper change. Are you keeping him up for more than fifteen or twenty minutes after daytime feedings? Even though he may seem to be wide awake, he doesn't really have the stamina to last much longer. You shouldn't wait for him to fall asleep before you put him down. Are you allowing him to become overstimulated by taking him with you when you run errands? Is he being overhandled by strangers (i.e., anyone other than grandparents)? These are things that can tire him out and make him colicky.

Gas. You might expect that because nursing is the more natural way to feed your baby, that it would also lead to fewer gassy episodes. Unfortunately, this isn't always the case. If you are a bountiful milk producer and/or your breasts let down forcefully, there may be feedings that start so quickly that your baby feels like he is drowning. Faced with this geyser of milk, he must decide if he is going to allow this mixture of fluid and air into his lungs or his stomach. Wisely, he chooses the latter but then must figure out what to do with the air. If he isn't able to burp it all out, it may come back to haunt him later as gas pains. This phenomenon seems to be more common when mothers have nursed a previous child or children, but many first-time nursing mothers who have an overly vigorous let-down reflex experience it, too.

Eventually your baby will learn to manage the flow of milk and/or burp more efficiently. However, this may take as long as three months. Happily there are a few things that you can try in an effort to improve the situation in the meantime. First, review your burping technique (see Appendix 1). Second, burp your baby four or five minutes into the feeding instead of waiting until he has finished on one breast. Babies naturally swallow more air at the beginning of the feeding as they create suction. If not burped out, this gas will be pushed from his stomach into his intestines by the flow of milk. Once it has passed out of his stomach, it can't be removed by burping and may cause pain later in the day.

If you find that your initial flow of milk is too forceful for your baby, hand-express or pump for a minute or two before you put him to your breast. In another two or three weeks this extra step will no longer be necessary as he learns to manage your let-down reflex.

You can try to give your baby simethicone drops. This over-the-counter medication is intended to convert large gas bubbles into smaller ones. It is safe and without significant side effects. Unfortunately, it is seldom terribly effective. Try giving your baby

0.4 cc with each daytime feeding. To be effective at all, it must be taken when the air is being swallowed. It won't work if your baby is already having a gas pain. If you don't notice any improvement after finishing a bottle of the stuff, don't bother buying another. On the other hand, if it does seem to help, you can continue to give it for months if necessary.

It is unlikely that your diet is contributing to your baby's gassiness, but review the section on the relationship between your breast milk and what you eat on page 140. The timing of the feeding may be causing a problem. Some scientists believe that the last milk to leave your breast (known as hindmilk) is richer than that produced in the first half of the feeding (foremilk). If your baby has become accustomed to feeding on only one side at a time, he may be receiving a larger dose of hindmilk than he can comfortably digest. The solution is to shorten his feeding to five minutes on the first side so that he will be forced to feed on the second side. If he wants more, then return him to the first side for another five minutes and then the second side, continuing to alternate until he is satisfied. This strategy will help limit the amount of hindmilk that he ingests.

Many babies swallow large amounts of air and pass it without any apparent discomfort. Why other babies seem to be so troubled by gas is not clear. However, I suspect that many of these colicky babies are more sensitive to the pain because they are also overtired. In my experience, the most successful management of colic is a combination of paying close attention to both gas management and sleep.

19

WEEK FOUR: ADJUSTING TO THE NEW REALITY

It's time for your baby's one-month checkup and another chance to see how you're doing. If things seem to have been going well, you may not have spoken to the pediatrician in the last three weeks. On the other hand, you may have made multiple trips into the office to reassure yourself that your baby is still gaining. In that case the one-month well-child checkup is yet another opportunity to make sure that your baby is healthy and that you are making enough milk.

Like most mothers you probably have a pretty good idea that you are meeting your baby's nutritional needs based on your own observation that he seems contented after nearly every feeding. However, there are some babies who don't complain appropriately if they are being shortchanged. As long as they are hugged and cuddled, they don't seem to mind that they have finished the day a few calories short. These eternal optimists will continue to lose weight without a whimper. In fact they may begin to sleep longer as they become weaker.

If the pediatrician feels that your baby is not gaining weight adequately, she may merely suggest that you feed more often or longer and return in a week or two for another weight check. Usually, more frequent, rather than longer, nursings are the better answer. This may mean tinkering with your baby's sleep schedule by waking him after three or four hours for a feeding if he doesn't wake on his own. Obviously, this sort of tampering is not something that you will want to do unless the pediatrician thinks it is absolutely necessary. If your baby is contented and gaining, but not quite enough to make the doctor happy, question if waking is really necessary. Ask if she thinks it would be safe to leave things as they are and come in for another weight check in a week.

On the other hand, if your baby is losing weight, the pediatrician is likely to suggest that you begin to supplement with formula. This is good advice if you are already nursing so often that you are exhausted. However, if your baby's sleep intervals are longer than four hours, you may ask if you can wake your baby more often and/or pump during those longer intervals to see if you can boost your milk production over the next week.

If you and the pediatrician decide to offer formula, it is okay to use a bottle at this point, but always give it *after* an attempt at nursing. This will help keep your baby interested in your breast. Begin by offering it no more often than once after every other feeding. This strategy is less likely to jeopardize the breastfeeding because it will encourage your baby to go to the breast often. This period of supplementation may be temporary. After a week or two, your milk supply may improve and the formula may be unnecessary. This is particularly true if you are still recovering from an unusually difficult delivery or have been sick or anemic.

Some mothers may need to supplement indefinitely to keep their babies growing adequately. There is nothing wrong with this arrangement. It may not be the way we had planned or hoped to feed your baby, but we've got to do what we've got to do. Remember, this isn't a competition. We want you to have a healthy and happy baby who has a healthy and happy mother. If that means that your baby's diet is 40 percent or even 70 percent formula, that's just the way it will be. The way you feed your baby is only a small part of parenting.

At the one-month visit the pediatrician will also examine your baby to make sure that all organ systems are developing on schedule. He may receive a shot, but it is usually not an immunization that causes much reaction. Ask the pediatrician to explain what you can expect.

Infrequent bowel movements . . . it happens. Up to this point you have become accustomed to changing anywhere from three to eight messy diapers every day. There may have been some stretches during which it seemed that every feeding was punctuated with the explosive rumble that announced that there was another mustard-like bowel movement to clean up. At around one month of age many breastfed babies begin to skip days between bowel movements. The first time this occurs it may worry you, but as long as your baby seems comfortable, is voiding frequently, and is gaining weight, you needn't be concerned.

As far as I know there is no scientific explanation for this decrease in frequency. Just think of it as a normal, unheralded benefit of breastfeeding. It is not unusual for a nursing baby to go a week between bowel movements, and I have known at least two breastfed infants who have regularly gone two weeks between bowel movements. However, don't forget that *before* a month of age infrequent bowel movements may be a sign that your milk supply is inadequate.

You may notice that your baby begins to act a bit uncomfortable and feed less vigorously for a few hours before he has a bowel movement, but as long as his discomfort is less than half a day, I urge you to avoid helping him along with invasive measures such as a rectal thermometer or suppositories. As long as he has not been drinking any formula, the stools themselves will continue to be loose and easy to pass even if it has been many days since the previous bowel movement.

On the other hand, if you have been using a formula supplement, some of the bowel movements may be firm and your baby my have to strain a bit to pass them. This is to be expected, and your baby has the coordination and strength to do it. If the process goes on for hours or the bowel movements are so hard that they cause bleeding, you may want to consider giving your baby some apple juice as a laxative. Start with regular pasteurized adult (not baby) apple juice mixed with an equal part water. An ounce of this mixture once or twice a day is usually sufficient. Be careful not to overdose him because you may create more discomfort than he started with in the form of gas cramps and diarrhea. If the apple juice doesn't help, consult your pediatrician for other remedies.

Growth spurts. Helping your baby learn sleep independence is a gradual and not always steady process. After a few weeks of sleeping at least three or four hours between nighttime feedings, your baby may begin to wake every two hours. There may be several explanations for this disappointing phenomenon. It may simply be that your baby's body is growing and he needs more milk to sustain a growth spurt. More frequent feedings send a message to your body to produce more milk, and after a few days your baby will return to his previous and more tolerable schedule. If he doesn't, it may mean that for some reason your milk supply has dwindled or you are unable to keep up. This is very unlikely, but you should consider taking your baby back to the pediatrician's office to be weighed. Is he gaining adequately? Are *you* healthy? Do you feel ill? Have you been trying to do too much? If you have allowed yourself to become overtired, your milk supply will suffer.

If your baby is beginning to wake frequently but doesn't seem terribly hungry, he may be ill or overtired. Have you been careful to keep his days mellow? Are you taking him out to the grocery store too often or having too many visitors? If you can't explain his fussiness, it is probably time for another trip to the pediatrician.

Are you happy? Episodes of sadness are extremely common in the first few months after delivery. Somewhere between 50 and 70 percent of new mothers will experience these "baby blues." Some days you may find yourself crying about things that don't usually upset you. Although you may have eagerly anticipated the birth of your baby, it's probably more work than you expected. In fact you may not find much in your life that makes you happy.

Some researchers have found that these unhappy thoughts are more likely to occur to breastfeeding mothers, but others see no such association. However, it is clear that women who have had a history of depression prior to becoming pregnant are much more likely to have postpartum depression. In my experience another important factor is fatigue. Mothers who can't get enough sleep—whether they are nursing or bottle feeding—are much more likely to become depressed. This is one of the reasons that I urge you to keep your schedule light and to avoid becoming your baby's pacifier.

At this point you should still be trying to nap whenever your baby is sleeping in order to repay the sleep debt that you will inevitably incur during night feedings. You can also use your baby's naps to get out of the house for a little sun and fresh air. Ask someone from your support group to come over and watch the baby for an hour so that you can get outside to enjoy a little of nature's own antidepressants—sunshine and some light exercise.

If more sleep and fresh air don't help, talk to your doctor about antidepressant medication. In the last few years several antidepressants have been determined to be safe and effective and are commonly prescribed, including Prozac among others. Although the FDA may not have officially approved Prozac for lactating women, thousands of women, including some in my own practice, have used it and other antidepressants safely and successfully while nursing. Some of these medications have been available for relatively short periods of time, so no one can absolutely guarantee that they will be harmless for your infant. However, the benefits of breastfeeding for the first three months easily outweigh the small risk of side effects associated with antidepressants. If you feel medication could help, discuss the issue carefully with your physician. If she seems unwilling to even consider prescribing medication while you are breastfeeding, you may want to seek a second opinion.

THE BOTTLE

It's time to introduce a bottle. A month ago you were struggling against the temptation to take the easy way out and give your baby a bottle. At the time nipple confusion could have sent the breastfeeding plan into a tailspin. Four weeks later it's a whole new ball game. He knows that your nipple is where the good stuff comes from, and he is taking enough of it to grow and stay contented. If you have any plans to continue nursing your baby when you go back to work, someone is going to give him at least one or two bottles each day. If your baby can learn to accept a bottle now, that will be one less sticky transition to negotiate when your maternity leave is over.

Breast milk should be the first thing that you offer in a bottle. It has a familiar taste and you know that your baby can digest it easily. I'm often asked if I have a favorite nipple to recommend. The short answer is: I don't. Each company claims that its latex or silicone nipple most closely resembles the natural shape or texture of a human nipple. But let's face it, your baby can't read the advertisements, and he will choose whichever nipple suits his fancy. You may have to buy several different ones before you find one that he will take.

Timing the first bottle may be a bit tricky. Of course your baby will be more receptive if he is hungry. However, if he is too hungry, he may also be too impatient to put up with any experimentation. Fill the first bottle with just a couple of ounces because he will likely balk at this new approach, and there is no sense wasting precious breast milk. Once you can count on him taking a bottle, he will probably take at least four ounces, but be prepared to give him six if he still seems hungry. Allow him to drink as much as he will take in a twenty-minute period, but there is no need to give him more than eight ounces in a single bottle.

It is very likely that your baby will refuse a bottle from you because he expects you to give him your breast. If this is the case, see if he's more receptive to a bottle from Dad or another familiar face. If you are lucky and your baby accepts a bottle without much complaint, I suggest that you continue to offer him a bottle every two or three days so that the bottle becomes a familiar alternative.

If your first few tries at bottle feeding are a complete bust, keep plugging away, offering a bottle every two or three days. However, if each attempt degenerates into a battle that ends in a sweaty screaming fit, stop. While unfortunate, it's not the end of the world. When you go back to work, your baby will quickly learn that when you're not there, he will have to get his food from some other source. Trust me, he will not starve. It may be an unpleasant day and a half for the daycare provider, but in the end your baby *will* take a bottle. In Chapter 21 you will read how to make this process go more smoothly, but for now don't fret about it. Enjoy the next two months of breastfeeding. We'll cross this bridge when we come to it.

If you are not planning on going back to work, but would like to leave your baby with someone else for just a few hours, see the discussion later in this chapter. Even if your baby refuses a bottle, there are still ways to get out of the house without nursing in public.

Is it time to start pumping and storing milk? In my experience most nursing mothers find pumping one of the less pleasant parts of their breastfeeding experience, and you probably don't want to rush into it before you have to. That said, it is a good idea to pump and save sixteen ounces of breast milk to be used in case you need to be away for a few hours sometime in the next month or two, even if you aren't planning to continue nursing when you go back to work. This will allow you to leave without having to worry how your baby will digest formula for the first time.

If you hope to keep breastfeeding when you return to your job and you want to avoid exposing your baby to formula, then you should probably start pumping and saving now so that your milk bank will be large enough to carry you through some almost inevitable lean times. Remember that the Maternity Leave Breastfeeding Plan is meant to be a realistic, family-friendly approach to nursing. If you find that pumping is an uncomfortable nuisance, or discover that you can pump only a few ounces at each sitting, you may want to rethink your plans to pump when you return to work. It may be more realistic to focus on enjoying these first three months and add formula, if necessary, when you go back to the job. Breast milk can be safely stored up to six months in your home freezer. If you have access to a commercial grade "deep freezer" (-20°F), you can store your milk for twelve months. Once thawed to room temperature the breast milk should be discarded after twenty-four hours. Never refreeze it.

Although some lactation experts feel that freshly pumped breast milk can be safely used after sitting at room temperature for up to ten hours, I recommend you discard it after six hours. In your refrigerator it may be kept for up to twenty-four hours.

If you are unable to pump enough to make it worth the effort, don't feel that you are less than the perfect mother. In fact you are in the majority. Even with the best of equipment many, if not most, women I see in my practice have difficulty producing milk with the artificial stimulation of a pump. Although they have been able to nurse their babies successfully, the unnatural sensations and sounds produced by the mechanical pump make it difficult for them to relax and let down. So while I encourage you to try pumping and storing, don't get depressed or feel inadequate if it doesn't work.

Leaking breasts. Although by this time your baby's demand for milk and your body's milk production schedule should have reached an equilibrium, you may be one of those unfortunate women whose breasts leak milk at awkward moments. Many mothers find that it if they hear their baby, or in some cases any baby, cry, their milk will let down. Other women need only think about their baby to saturate their blouses with milk. Unfortunately, reliable remedies for these damp disasters are scarce. Dark clothing and absorbent pads are your best bets. Make sure that you change pads frequently to protect your nipples from skin irritation and infection. Some mothers have found that firm pressure on their breasts with the flat of their hands can stem the flow. Do not try to adjust your milk supply by limiting your fluid intake because you may overcorrect and leave your baby with less milk than his body demands.

PUTTING THE PIECES BACK TOGETHER

Let's face it, once you have a baby your life will never be the same. You still weigh fifteen pounds more than your prepregnancy weight. Your only regular exercise consists of climbing the stairs to retrieve a forgotten diaper. You haven't had your hair cut in months, and you can't remember the last time you and your husband shared a bottle of wine over a candlelit dinner.

There just hasn't been time or energy to begin the rebuilding process. But it has been a month since you delivered and the nursing is going well enough that you can at least think about resuming some of your favorite activities. However, don't rush the process. Your body is still recovering, and you are still responsible for nourishing another human being, one that is growing rapidly. Your baby needs calories (a measure of energy) and you are the source. Even if you've been careful to avoid becoming a pacifier and are napping whenever you can, there may not be enough energy left over to do all the things you want to do. So take it easy. Rome wasn't built in a day.

Dropping a few pounds. Although you will feel much more like your old prematernal self if you could just drop a few pounds, I urge you to avoid dieting while you are nursing. It is difficult to calculate how many calories you must consume to keep up your milk supply, and I have known several mothers who have brought their nursing careers to a premature end by limiting their diets. Some well-known weight-loss programs suggest that breastfeeding women can safely follow their meal plans by adding a certain number of calories to their daily allotment. However, I think we don't understand enough about the biology of human milk production to make these suggestions compatible with nursing.

There is a poorly understood correlation between how much fat you eat and the fat content of your milk. What is clear is that if you restrict your fat intake too much, you may jeopardize the quality of your milk. Remember, fat isn't always bad. In fact your baby needs fat in his diet to build a healthy body, particularly a nervous system.

The best thing you can do for your body at this point is to eat a healthy, varied diet that is heavy on the fruits and vegetables and light on the baked goods. Begin some light aerobic exercise to tone up the muscles that haven't been doing much work for the last seven or eight months. You may lose a few pounds, but more important you will begin to feel better. If you plan to stop nursing after three months, you have only two more months before you can take a more aggressive approach to weight loss. Even if you decide to nurse longer, your baby will get enough nutrition from solid foods by the time he is six or seven months old, that you could safely begin to carefully limit your caloric intake then. If your milk supply begins to diminish at that time, he will usually be able to make up the difference with solids.

Regardless of when you begin to diet, do it gradually and with the advice of your physician or a certified nutritionist. If you are still nursing, make sure that your baby is weighed by the pediatrician regularly and make periodic appointments with your own physician. Even if he is getting solid food, you and/or your baby may become undernourished if you have cut back your intake of calories too drastically.

Getting back in shape. If you were accustomed to regular aerobic exercise before becoming pregnant, you are probably itching to get back to your health club or to pounding the pavement on your favorite three-mile loop around the neighborhood. Like most of us who work out regularly, you realize that in addition to making our body feel better, exercise is also a potent antidepressant. Fortunately breastfeeding and aerobic exercise are compatible. However, there are just a few things to consider before you go rummaging in the bottom of your closet for your running shoes.

First, there is the simple matter of the changes that have taken place in your body. You are out of shape and your breasts probably weigh twice as much as they did before you started nursing. Start by buying yourself a new sports bra. Begin your return to fitness slowly and take it easy. For example, walk half of your normal running route for the first few days. Then walk the whole route for a week, then jog half and walk half. You get the idea.

Once you are feeling fit enough to begin a vigorous workout, be careful to keep yourself well hydrated. Your breast milk is mostly water, and if you haven't replenished the fluid you lose as sweat, your milk supply may suffer. Exercise may also affect the taste of your milk. It turns out that when some women exercise vigorously, the lactic acid produced in their muscles can filter into their milk and give it a sour taste. This phenomenon is rare and most babies don't seem to mind breastfeeding after their mothers have exercised. However, if you notice that your baby doesn't like to nurse immediately after you have worked out, wait half an hour to an hour. This will give your body's circulatory system time to clear the lactic acid from your breasts. There is no need to pump and discard the milk you have made while you were exercising.

At one to two months of age your baby is probably too young to accompany you in a baby jogger if you plan to do anything more than a slow jog on smooth surfaces. Although I have never seen any scientific documentation of damage directly related to baby joggers, I think many pediatricians like myself are concerned about the shaking trauma that a two- or three-month-old baby might suffer.

I would also urge you to avoid a health-club nursery (or any other kind) for the first three months. Even though he is breastfed your baby is very vulnerable to infection, and a cold can be devastating. The last section in this chapter will give you some suggestions on how to get out of the house safely.

Is it safe to get a perm? A little exercise and some fresh air will go a long way toward making you feel like your old self. You'd feel even better if you could find the time to get your hair done. Don't let rumors about the danger of chemicals used to curl hair stop you. Somewhere many years ago a rumor began that the chemicals used to curl hair can render breast milk unsafe. I have searched for some scientific validation of this claim but can find none.

If your favorite hairstyle requires getting a permanent, do it. Don't worry that your baby will suffer some ill effects. I have never seen or heard of it happening. By the way, it is also safe to have dental X-rays. They will not adversely affect your milk.

Would you like a glass of wine? As soon as you discovered that you were pregnant, you probably swore off alcohol. While the evidence supporting total abstinence during pregnancy may still be a bit shaky, I think your decision to avoid alcohol was a good one. Should you still decline the offer of a glass of wine or beer now that you are nursing? Scientific data regarding this question is even more murky. My answer has always been that as far as we know a single glass of wine or beer when consumed with a meal will not cause any lasting harm to your nursing baby.

Some people may warn you that your baby may be more sleepy if he has feasted on alcohol-tainted milk. However, I recently read an article in a medical journal that suggested just the opposite. During the three and a half hours following a feeding of alcohol-containing milk, the babies in this study spent significantly less time sleeping than when they had been fed alcohol-free milk. So far no one has explained this phenomenon. Unless you notice that your baby sleeps less well after you have had a drink, don't worry about it.

There is also scant scientific evidence to support the old wives' tale that drinking beer will increase your milk supply. In fact some researchers feel that more than a small amount of alcohol may actually decrease your milk production. If you tend to be very tense and have trouble relaxing when you feed your baby, a glass of beer (or wine) before a feeding may help you let down. This is not a recommendation to toss down a six-pack every day. The old adage of "everything in moderation" couldn't be more true than when it is applied to your diet during breastfeeding.

Getting out of the house. Even if you're not craving some aerobic exercise, you are probably eager to get out of the house to see what the rest of the world has been up to while you were busy having and then feeding your baby. Here in Maine we call that urge cabin fever, and while the desire won't make your temperature rise, it can certainly make you crazy.

There are several solutions. The most obvious is to take your baby with you for a short walk around the neighborhood. If your baby is just a month or two old, he will still be vulnerable to temperature extremes, so if the temperature is less than 60°F, or more than 90°F, you shouldn't take him outside for anything more than a quick run to the car. He should be protected from the wind and direct sun. Those old-fashioned baby carriages with high sides and a hood are excellent examples of the kind of protection your young infant needs.

You must also be wary of curious neighbors and small children. Although your baby receives some protective antibodies in your breast milk, he is still vulnerable to illness, including the common cold. If you are unable to keep strangers and curious neighbors out of his face, you may have to reconsider your decision, or at least the timing, of your plan to walk around the neighborhood.

Remember that you are still trying to teach your baby how to put himself to sleep. A trip outside must be carefully scheduled into his day so it doesn't disturb the sleep patterns you are trying to instill. In his first two or three months your baby simply may not have the time to squeeze in a walk between naps and feedings. If, however, he is well on his way toward sleep independence and will sleep in his stroller, a walk might take the place of one of his naps.

Don't despair if your baby's sleep schedule won't allow him to venture out of the house. You can ask or hire someone to watch him while you go out yourself. Your first choice will probably be your husband, but I suspect that someone from your support team will be more than happy to watch your baby for an hour or two. You may feel ambivalent about your first venture out of the house without him. On the one hand, you desperately want some time for yourself, but on the other you worry that your baby won't be safe or comfortable in someone else's care. All of this is normal. It will take time and there may be several false starts before you can do it.

Start with a modest separation of an hour or less and build up gradually. At this point your baby's longest daytime feeding interval is probably no more than four hours, and so it would be unwise to plan a longer outing. Even the most experienced baby-sitter will feel uncomfortable if you have not left at least one bottle of breast milk or formula. Remind them that this is to be used only for an emergency such as a flat tire that might delay your expected return. Hopefully, you'll feed your baby just before you leave. Reassure the sitter that even if you aren't back for twelve hours, the baby is not going to starve. If the baby gets fussy, ask the sitter to hold off feeding the baby if it has been less than three hours since his last feeding. Unfortunately, some baby-sitters will reach for the bottle at the baby's first whimper. A just-fed baby may take some milk despite his full stomach and then the sitter must deal with the vomiting.

Make sure that if you plan on leaving a formula bottle, your baby has successfully taken and digested formula before. You don't want him to have a bad reaction to a new food while you are away.

Provide the sitter with an accurate prediction of when you plan to return home, and tell her that both you and your baby would rather wait for a breastfeeding. If he seems to want to eat and there will be only thirty or forty-five minutes until your expected return, instruct the sitter to try her best to comfort him by walking around. Reassure her that hunger isn't going to hurt him. When you arrive your breasts will be more than ready to comfort him and he will forgive and forget. Offer to pay her time and a half for that fussy period, because she, and not the baby, will undoubtedly be more uncomfortable.

Although it is not the option I prefer, you can bring the baby with you when you leave the house and nurse him if he gets hungry. Even if the thought of nursing in public doesn't bother you, I suggest you wait another three or four weeks before you begin to consider taking the baby out of the house for anything more than a quick trip to Grandma's house. I have already warned you about the risk of infection and the likelihood that schedule disruptions may make your baby fussy. By the time your child is entering his third month, these two issues are less of a problem. At the end of the next chapter you will find a section about the art of nursing in public.

Sex. Although your husband may have been eager to resume your sexual relationship two weeks ago, intercourse may still not be high on your list. Eventually it will, and you must be prepared with some form of contraception. Remember, it is risky and unwise to count on breastfeeding as a form of birth control.

There are birth control pills compatible with nursing, and obviously, barrier contraception such as condoms and diaphragms will not affect your breast milk. Discuss your options with your obstetrician.

It is not unusual for your breasts to leak during sexual arousal or stimulation. Rest assured that the amount of milk lost is not significant, at least as far as your baby is concerned.

20

THE SECOND MONTH: STRIKING
A BALANCE

While I can't guarantee that you will enjoy nursing every day, I do believe that after navigating the difficult first week or two, most women are happy with their decision to breastfeed. If after four weeks nursing isn't meeting the expectations I described in Chapter 9, I apologize for leading you astray. But before you decide to pack it in and switch to formula, please give it a few more weeks. There are better things ahead, and this chapter will help you begin to strike a balance in your life. Until now, nursing may have felt like your sole occupation. The next few pages will show how you can move beyond your role as a milk machine and begin to feel like a human being again.

Creating order out of chaos. I hope that you are more rested than you were a month ago, and I trust that you have been able to pick up a few of the pieces of your old life with your new baby, though life probably remains chaotic. Most feedings are followed by a quiet play period and, thanks to your determination to not become a pacifier, the baby falls asleep when you put him in his crib most of the time. But intervals between feedings are still unpredictable. It is hard to get anything accomplished around the house or plan a jogging date with a friend because you aren't sure whether your baby's next sleep interval will last two hours or four.

Don't worry. Mother Nature is on your side and things will get better if we are patient. For biologic reasons that we still don't understand, your baby will begin to drop feedings and continue to gain wait. By the time he is four months old he could be down to just six feedings a day. At six months he may be down to four. The amazing thing is that these few remaining feedings won't seem to take any longer than when he was nursing more often. Somehow you and he will have become dramatically more efficient.

The process by which your baby drops feedings will occur more quickly if you have been careful to avoid becoming a pacifier. The unfortunate mother who has allowed herself to become a mandatory component of her baby's sleep ritual will still be participating in many sleep-related "feedings" or snacks that your baby will have already given up.

Unfortunately, even if you have been careful to guide your baby toward sleep independence, I can't guarantee that you will be free of middle-of-the-night feedings anytime soon. Some babies simply can't go longer than six hours without getting hungry. It's possible your six or seven month old may continue to wake and feed vigorously for fifteen or twenty minutes at 2 A.M., even though he may be getting solids two or three times a day and be perfectly capable of putting himself to sleep. The good news is that these night feedings shouldn't take more than half an hour. By the time your child is nine months old night feedings will have disappeared with or without your tinkering.

Although the decline in total number of feedings will eventually help make your days run more smoothly, the next section describes some things to do that will make your life less chaotic.

Should you put your baby on a schedule or feed "on demand"? The answer is both. Let me explain: It is unreasonable to expect your six-week-old infant to feed on a regular three- or four-hour schedule of your design. It just won't work. It is like trying to fit a square peg into a round hole. There are too many variables driving his hunger and your milk production to expect a strict schedule to be successful.

On the other hand, when parents indefinitely feed their baby "on demand" the chaos typical of the first few weeks often continues for months longer than necessary. The problem is that some parents interpret every cry and whimper as a "demand" for food. Babies cry for a variety of reasons. They cry when they are uncomfortable, they cry when they are hungry, and very often they cry when they are tired. Many babies will refuse to be fed if they aren't hungry, but some babies will continue to suckle because it makes them feel better even though the real problem is that they have a wet diaper or are tired. Babies who have been allowed to use their mother's breasts (or a bottle) as a sleep aid will feed although their primary problem is fatigue and not hunger. The extra milk they receive during these nonnutritive feedings will either be vomited up later on, or accumulate as rings of baby fat around ankles and wrists. Yes, breastfed babies can become overweight.

The solution to this dilemma is what might be called a flexible schedule. By now you should be able to identify your baby's tired cry, but if you still have one leg in the pacifier trap, turn to Chapter 18. To create a flexible schedule start by renewing your commitment to the "I will not become a pacifier!" credo.

You should continue to nurse your baby when his "demand" is for food. However, if a "feeding" lasts for only a few minutes, refuse to offer him your breast the next time a similar situation arises. Say your baby wakes up at midnight for two or three nights in a row but only feeds for three or four minutes before falling back to sleep. Don't rush in to nurse him the next time that he cries at midnight. The fact is, we all have short awakenings throughout the night as our bodies' sleep cycles ebb and flow. Babies have more of these "arousals," particularly if they are over-tired, and will put themselves back to sleep if given the opportunity to do so. However, if you continue to nurse your baby even though hunger wasn't the cause of his arousal, he will continue to expect you to participate in the process night after night after night.

The best solution is to assign your husband the job of dealing with these nonhunger-related wakenings. Your baby won't expect his father to nurse him and will realize more quickly that his only option is to go back to sleep. Whoever draws the short straw to check on the baby should do as little as possible to quiet the crying before returning him to his crib while he is still awake. The more you do, the more your child will expect the next time he wakes. Remember, your baby can learn to put himself to sleep if you give him the chance. This tactic is at the heart of the sleep-management strategy that was made famous by Dr. Richard Ferber in the 1980s. Don't turn on the light, don't take your baby out of his bedroom, and above all remember that your goal is to calm your baby down, not to put him to sleep. Even if the baby begins to cry as soon as you return him to his crib, leave the room and wait a few minutes longer than you did the first time before reentering the room and repeating the process. If two hours have passed since the first arousal, feed him and try again the next night. Remember that this advice about "Ferberization" applies only to the situations in which you are confident that your baby is not waking because he is hungry. A more detailed discussion of sleep management is available in my book *Is My Child Overtired?* (Simon & Schuster, 2000).

Building a routine. Babies and small children find the predictability of a schedule comforting. They thrive on a routine, and now is the time to begin building one for your baby. For the first month or so your baby's biologic needs drove your family's schedule, but now it is your turn to take the leadership role. I am not suggesting that you impose an arbitrary four-hour feeding schedule on him—it seldom works, anyway. What I am proposing is that you begin introducing some consistent elements into the activities that you and your baby do together. If you have followed my suggestions about a "lights out" routine from seven at night until seven in the morning, you have already begun the process. Now add things like baths, walks to the mailbox, and reading books to the routine. For example, your baby's schedule might include "lights on" at 7 A.M., bath at 9 A.M., walk around the neighborhood at 3 P.M., and "lights out" at 7 P.M. Obviously, your decision about where to insert these activities will be based on previous observations of when your baby seems to be most alert.

Gradually, your baby's feeding and napping schedule will begin to fall into step with this primitive routine, and you will discover that you have more time for yourself. At the very least the time you have is more predictable. When it is time for you to return to your job the routine will be more fully developed and with some minor tinkering we can adapt it your work schedule.

Nursing strikes. In the last chapter I warned you that your baby may suddenly begin to nurse more frequently in an attempt to build up your milk production. A less common phenomenon is often referred to as a nursing strike. Without warning, your infant may decide he doesn't like to nurse. If this happens, look for signs of illness and consult the pediatrician. She will want to examine him and will pay particular attention to his mouth to make sure that he can still suck and swallow comfortably.

If your baby seems healthy, think carefully about things that may affect your milk supply. Has illness, fatigue, or dehydration caused a decrease in your milk production? If your menstrual period has recently begun again, this may be associated in a temporary dip in your milk supply. Although most babies will want to nurse *more* often when you aren't providing enough milk, some will decide that you aren't worth the effort and go on strike. It doesn't make much sense, but it happens. If you suspect this is the case, pump frequently, eat and drink well, and get plenty of rest. Hopefully your supply will return in a day or two and your baby will nurse vigorously again.

Some apparently healthy babies take a dislike to breastfeeding despite having mothers who are consistent and bountiful producers. I suspect that in a few cases the child has been turned off by the taste of something in his mother's diet that has seeped into her milk, but in most cases the phenomenon defies explanation. Fortunately, most babies who go on strike eagerly return to their mother's breast before the week is out. If you are faced with this situation, continue to pump to maintain your supply. Be patient. Offer your pumped milk in a bottle if necessary and use formula only as a last resort. Keep in close contact with the pediatrician to make sure that your baby is still healthy. Unfortunately, some obstinate babies will steadfastly refuse to nurse again no matter how long you wait. You must then decide if you want to continue to pump so that your baby can still receive your breast milk. I have found that most mothers faced with a situation in which they receive no physical reward for their efforts can keep pumping for only a couple of weeks before their supply diminishes or the pumping gets old and tiresome. I don't blame them, nor will I blame you, for calling it quits. Raising your child should be fun. It wasn't your fault that your baby went on strike; you gave it your best shot.

Nursing in public . . . only if you want to. Now that you and your baby are an accomplished breastfeeding team, you can begin to think about taking the show on the road. If you feel comfortable nursing with strangers around, you will be able to venture out of the house with your baby free of worry that your excursion will be cut short by his feeding schedule. However, I hope I have made it clear that it is your baby's sleep requirements and not his hunger that should dictate his itinerary. At two or three months of age he should still be sleeping most of the time between feedings, and if, like the majority of infants, he sleeps best in his own crib, you both will be happier if you keep his public appearances short and timed to coincide with his usual awake periods. If you ignore his sleep needs when you plan your errands and social visits, your baby's cranky behavior later that day (and/or night) should remind you that you have overestimated his stamina. Of course there are babies who seem to sleep well anywhere and anytime, but they are the blessed few. Just because your five-month-old niece can sleep in the shopping cart at the grocery store and return home bubbly and cheerful doesn't mean that your child will be able to do the same.

Although you may feel comfortable nursing your baby in public, there are large segments of the population who would prefer you didn't. For them breastfeeding is an activity with sexual and biologic overtones that make them uncomfortable. While this attitude is gradually becoming less prevalent, it is not likely to disappear any time soon. In keeping with the reality-based premise of *The Maternity Leave Breastfeeding Plan*, I suggest that you be discreet when nursing in public. To do otherwise is to invite reactions that may be counterproductive, particularly if you are planning to continue nursing after you return to work. Some of your co-workers may already be ambivalent about nursing and the sight of your exposed breast may be enough to permanently remove them from your list of allies in your struggle to keep nursing.

Simply put, breastfeeding in twenty-first-century America can be hard enough, so it doesn't make sense to make it any more difficult for yourself by offending people whose attitudes are parochial and wrong.

The techniques of discreet breastfeeding are obvious. Choose clothing that can easily be lifted, unbuttoned, unsnapped, or unzipped to give your baby access to the nipple without exposing your entire breast. Many mothers also drape a blanket or shawl over their baby while he is feeding. In addition to creating the illusion that you really aren't nursing, it helps shield your baby from the distractions and hubbub around you. This will be particularly important as your child gets older and more curious.

If like many of us you're shy about your body, and don't feel comfortable breastfeeding in public, you still have plenty of options. At this age your baby should be able to fast for three or four hours before he *needs* to be fed, though he may *want* to be fed long before that. He may make your outing unpleasant because you aren't nursing him when he thinks it is time, but as long as you are planning on feeding him within four hours of his previous feeding, you aren't being cruel by making him wait.

While we all feel that we should stamp out hunger in the underprivileged third world countries, the kind of hunger your baby endures while he waits for thirty or forty minutes, until you can find a private place to breastfeed, is only an inconvenience and he will forgive and forget.

Obviously, you can minimize the chances that your trip out of the house will be interrupted by your baby's hunger by feeding him just before you leave home—after, for example, you are all dressed with makeup on and tote bag and diaper bag ready to go. Of course if your baby is flexible enough to accept an occasional bottle, you are all set. Even if he has refused a bottle in the past, it wouldn't hurt to bring one along. If he is truly hungry or thirsty, he will drink from a bottle. You needn't feel guilty if you have made the nipple hole large enough so that he can feel the sweet wetness of your breast milk on his lips and still stubbornly refuses to drink.

Second thoughts . . . sometimes they're the best. You may have decided to follow the Maternity Leave Breastfeeding Plan because you knew long before you became pregnant that you wanted to nurse for only a few months. However, now that you have been doing it for just over a month, you are surprised how much you like it. Some of your initial hesitation may have been a fear of failure. Now that you know you can breastfeed, there is a growing part of you that wants to keep going three months and beyond. You can't describe the feeling, but using your own body to feed your baby makes you feel good, good enough that you're willing to tackle the challenge of continuing when you go back to work. It is not too late to begin preparing for this option. Go back and read the section on how to create a nursing-friendly workplace. Listen to your body. If it is saying "Go for it!" why not give it a try? This book will support your effort, and I, for one, won't get on your case if you eventually decide it's just too much to handle.

On the other hand you may have been planning to continue nursing when you returned to work but now realize breastfeeding is taking far more energy than you anticipated. It may be time to reconsider your decision. There is no rush. You probably still have a month and a half or two before you will go back to your job. Things are going to get better. In a few weeks your baby will be nursing less often, and you'll be getting more sleep. Your body is still in the process of recovering from delivery, particularly if you bled enough to become anemic.

If two months from now things are better, but breastfeeding is still taking too great a toll on your body or it just isn't much fun, then you should stop. I wrote this book because many women find that combining work and breastfeeding is just too exhausting. Go back and read Chapter 5. It will help you realize that how you feed your baby is just one small part of parenting. Your baby will love you just as much if you decide to give him formula when you go back to work.

Accept those second thoughts as normal—because they are. Enjoy these next months before it's time to go back to work. Don't worry about what your sister who is still nursing her two year old will think. Eventually, she will understand that there is more than one correct way to raise a child.

21

THE THIRD MONTH: ENJOYING YOUR BABY AND MAKING TRANSITIONS

By this time you and your baby should be a skilled and efficient nursing team. Most feedings come at predictable times and are less frequent than they were a month ago. You may be nursing only five or six times in twenty-four hours. You should have more time to yourself because your baby is taking naps at least an hour and a half long, and he is probably sleeping five or six hours at a stretch at night.

You may still get tired from time to time—after all, you're a parent—but you should have much more stamina than you did six weeks ago. Most important, you should be enjoying this time at home with your baby. Every day he is doing something new. His personality is emerging. He can recognize you from across the room. He not only smiles but laughs. Although he lacks intelligible words, the two of you can hold long conversations about almost anything.

However, there is darkness on the horizon. In thirty days you will be returning to work and this will mean either weaning or dealing with the hassle of pumping. Neither alternative feels very appealing at this point, but don't let your concerns about what is going to happen next month distract you from enjoying the next month at home with your baby.

Remember that one of the reasons that you spent so much time and energy trying to make your workplace nursing-friendly before you delivered was so that you could enjoy this last month at home. Of course there are unknowns. There always will be, but please don't allow them to dampen your enthusiasm for nursing just as you and your baby are getting good at it.

You can wait until just three or four days before you go back to work before you start the weaning process, if that is the path you have chosen. In fact you will probably still be nursing in the evenings and at night for a few weeks after you return to your job. You may discover that partial weaning works fine, and you will still be able to nurse part-time for several more months. So, with apologies to Yogi Berra, it may not be over when it's over. Regardless of when and how your breastfeeding career finishes, there is no sense in fretting about weaning now.

Even if your baby is one of those stubborn little buggers who hasn't accepted a bottle yet, don't worry. Necessity is still the mother of invention. Push will come to shove and in a day and a half your baby will be drinking from a bottle if you aren't around to nurse him. It may be an unpleasant day or two for the sitter, but your baby isn't going to starve, and the ugly part of the transition will be over before you know it.

PUMPING AND STORING YOUR MILK

Is pumping going to work? Although I have just encouraged you to pretend, at least for the moment, you aren't going to have to return to work, there is one critical issue that we can't ignore if you plan on continuing to breastfeed: pumping. I have devoted little space to this subject before now because I want you to enjoy as much of your breastfeeding experience as possible, and I think that most women would agree that pumping just isn't much fun. However, if you hope to accumulate a backup supply of breast milk that will give you some flexibility when you return to work, you should begin pumping now.

As I warned you way back in Chapter 9 there is no guarantee that you will be successful at pumping. not every woman is biologically capable of getting pregnant, not every woman who delivers a baby can make enough milk to fulfill her baby's nutritional needs, and not every woman who can successfully nurse her baby can extract enough milk from her breasts by artificial means (pumping or hand expression) to make the effort worthwhile.

Even with the best pump and under the most comfortable conditions some women find it difficult to extract a significant amount of milk from their breasts. What follows are some strategies that can make the artificial stimulation of a pump seem more natural, but I think we both must accept that these tricks don't work for everyone.

Make sure that you have a good pump. Of course any pump that works for you is a good pump, but in general the more you pay, the more likely you are to end up with an effective pump. Electric pumps are generally more efficient. You may want to replace the manual pump you bought when you planned on weaning at the end of your maternity leave. Will a pump system that offers a refrigerated storage compartment make things easier for you?

When is the best time to pump? There is no one best time to pump, but here are some options to consider. In the beginning you may be more successful if you pump one breast while your baby is nursing from the other one. The advantage of this strategy is that your body may be more likely to eject milk while you are hearing, seeing, and feeling the presence of your baby—all powerful stimuli. There are also disadvantages to this approach. The first is purely technical. Initially you may run out of hands as you attempt to cradle your baby and hold the pump at the same time. You endured similar fumbling when you started breastfeeding two months ago; it shouldn't be too long before you have mastered this more advanced technique. The second problem is that you may pump so much milk from that one breast that you short-change your baby when it's his turn. The solution is to start by pumping just for a few minutes with each feeding until your body senses the extra demand and begins producing more milk. If you are going to use this technique routinely, you should probably check with your pediatrician to make sure that your baby is continuing to gain weight.

If your baby has some predictable four-hour stretches between feedings, pumping two hours after a feeding will usually yield a significant amount of milk and still allow your body enough time to produce milk for your baby's next feeding. If he wakes unexpectedly, you can always offer him what you have just pumped if he doesn't seem satisfied with nursing.

Your most productive pumping sessions correspond with your baby's longest sleep intervals—generally at night. You will have to decide whether it is more important for you to get some sleep or build up your milk bank account. As you may have guessed from my previous suggestions about fatigue prevention, I encourage you to err on the side of getting more sleep and making up any milk shortfall by using formula. If you allow yourself to become exhausted by staying up at night to pump, you may run the risk of actually decreasing milk production.

What to do if you can pump only a few ounces at each sitting. First, don't worry that you actually aren't making enough milk for your baby. He is probably able to extract much more than you can pump. As long as he is gaining weight well, you are making plenty.

Make sure that you are keeping yourself well hydrated. If you are going to ask your body to make more milk, you must provide it with the raw materials. That means drinking an adequate amount of fluid and eating a healthy and abundant diet.

Create a relaxing environment in which you can pump. It should be private, quiet, and comfortable. Surround yourself with baby memorabilia. A picture of your infant, some of his clothes, even an audio- or videotape may help fool your mind and body into believing that the demand for milk is coming from your baby and not a mechanical pump.

Storing your milk. As long as you have been careful to use clean containers, your breast milk will keep safely in the refrigerator for twenty-four hours. If you have a reliable freezer, you can preserve your milk for six months (twelve months in a -20°F commercial freezer).

With experience you will hit upon the optimal size container. In general it is wise to store your milk in small quantities (four ounces or less). This will give you flexibility to match the vagaries in your child's appetite and minimize waste. Your breast milk is precious stuff.

Some of the pumping and/or bottle systems come with plastic bottle liners that can be used to store milk. Many mothers use small Ziploc-style bags, because their wide openings keep spillage to a minimum. Be sure to write the collection date on the containers and rotate your stock to avoid spoilage.

To thaw frozen milk place the container in hot tap water. Although a microwave might be quicker, microwave heat creates hot spots that could burn your baby's mouth and damage some of the nutritional components of the milk. Once the milk has been thawed it should be used promptly. It can be kept safely in the refrigerator for a few hours, but after that the risk of bacterial contamination increases. It should never be refrozen for reuse.

If despite your best efforts at creating the right atmosphere, you are able to pump only a few ounces, it is probably time to reevaluate your plan to continue nursing when you return to work. Unless you are able to bring your baby to work with you, or can find a daycare just a few minutes away, you will be forced to offer your baby formula while you are away. This is not the end of the world, and it may not even be the end of your nursing career. Your baby may continue to nurse when the two of you are together or he may decide that he would rather stick with the formula. If he chooses to stop nursing when you return to work, there isn't much you can do about it. Treasure the memories of your first three months together and remember that you have given him the best start possible.

If it is clear that pumping is not going to work, don't let this revelation ruin your last thirty days home together. Instead, enjoy the rest of your nursing experience. You don't need to start the transition back to work until the last week of your maternity leave.

THE TRANSITION WEEK

No matter when or how you do it, returning to work is going to be difficult. You can expect a tearful moment or two. Even though you have chosen his daycare carefully, it won't be easy to leave your baby in the care of people you just met a few times. Will they look after him as well as you have? Is he going to miss you? You know you are going to miss him.

To ease the transition, I suggest that you make it in gradual steps. This will allow you to iron out unforseeable wrinkles in your plan and give you a better chance to adjust psychologically to the separation. The whole process can be completed in less than a week. In fact three or four days is usually sufficient.

The first day your goal should be very modest—an hour at the office to reorganize your desk and have a cup of coffee with your fellow employees who will be eager to see the most recent pictures of your baby. Most moms seriously underestimate the time it takes to get themselves and their baby dressed, fed, and out of the house. If you are still nursing, you may decide to squeeze in two feedings before you leave the house, one as soon as your baby wakes and another just before you depart. Some mothers find that this second nursing is best done when they get to the daycare. If you have time for both feedings before you leave for work, there is a good chance that your baby may be able to make it all the way to lunch without another feeding. If you have been able to find daycare that is close enough to make lunchtimes with your baby practical, this arrangement may allow you to avoid bottles and formula.

Make the first day leisurely. There is no need to rush around.

You haven't promised to arrive at work on time, nor have you agreed to do any work. You are merely making a cameo appearance to get a rough idea of how your new schedule is going to work. The pressure to arrive on time will come soon enough.

After you have had a chance to reacquaint yourself with your fellow employees, head back to daycare. If your baby is sleeping, don't wake him. He is already beginning to build his own routine. Take the opportunity to go out and run a few errands, and return later to pick him up. Then go home and enjoy the rest of the day together.

If he has screamed the entire time you were at work, don't worry. Of course it is upsetting to discover that he was unhappy while you were away, but he will adjust to his new surroundings. An experienced daycare provider has seen it happen many times before and will reassure you that within a few days he will relax and accept the new status quo.

The second day you will have a more realistic idea of how early you will have to get up to arrive at work at the usual time. Plan to spend another hour or two at work before you leave to pick up your baby at lunchtime. Resist the temptation or urgings of your boss to stay longer or bring some work home to finish in the evening. Hopefully, you have negotiated some payment for these transition days, but regardless of whether you are getting paid, the goal of this first week is to make a smooth transition—not to get any significant amount of work done.

The next few days add another hour or two away from your baby. If staying around the office is awkward because there isn't much for you to do, use the time to shop, run errands, or get some exercise. Do not interrupt your baby's adjustment to the new schedule. If he is sleeping and enjoying himself, rejoice!

Although leaving the house in the morning may be chaotic the first few days, this should improve as you develop a more efficient routine. However, you may find that despite your best efforts, getting to work on time means getting up so early that you arrive at work exhausted and stressed. One solution is going to bed earlier. If that doesn't help, try negotiating a modified schedule that will allow more time in the morning to feed your baby. Hopefully, your boss knows what it's like to get an infant ready for the day.

Your first full day back at work. In a perfect world you would work part-time for the next three months. However, like most women, you will be returning to a full-time schedule after your short transition week. Even though we have done our best to minimize the emotional trauma to you and your baby by doing it gradually, you are bound to finish your first full day at work tired, tearful, and convinced—whether you continue to breastfeed or not—that you just won't have the stamina to work full-time, or even part-time, and be a mother.

Although your first day back at work may have been a logistical and emotional disaster, try not to let it depress you. Each day you will learn new strategies that will allow you to juggle motherhood and your career and still have some time for yourself at the end of the day. It will be a struggle in the beginning, but don't quit your job or give up breastfeeding until you have given your current arrangement a good week or two.

WHEN THE HANDWRITING ON THE WALL SAYS, "THIS ISN'T WORKING!"

I hope that by the end of your second week you feel that you have settled into a viable routine. By bedtime you run out of steam, but by the next morning you feel rested and ready to face the challenges that await. Your baby appears adjusted to his daycare and is happy to see you when you pick him up.

Unfortunately, not everyone's experience works out that way. By the beginning of your third week back at your job, you may find yourself struggling to get all of the puzzle pieces to fit. The combination of two or three night nursings and hectic days at the office may leave you feeling so tired in the morning that you are ready to climb back into bed after breakfast.

Your plan to pump at work may not be working out the way

you hoped it would. When you do have time, you are so fatigued and tense that you can barely pump three or four ounces. The supply of milk that you stored over the last month is dwindling because your body isn't able to keep up with the demand.

The truth is, this combination of working and nursing may not be feasible. Even if you heeded my warning about becoming a pacifier, even if you had succeeded in making your workplace nursing-friendly, even if your child was an eager and skillful nurser from day one, your body may simply decide that making milk for your baby is too much effort and shut down the supply.

If you aren't able to enjoy parenting because you have run out of both time and energy, something has got to change. This may happen despite your Maternity Leave Breastfeeding Plan working like a charm and meeting all of your expectations up to this point. You could continue to limp along and fantasize that your child will someday thank you for being a martyr for the cause of his nutrition, but likely he will never give it a thought. Unfortunately, there are women who continue to believe that martyrdom and motherhood are synonymous, and are more than willing to sacrifice their own happiness in pursuit of the title "super mom." Please don't allow yourself to fall into this trap. One of my goals in writing this book was to help more women truly enjoy their role as mothers.

Let's take a step back and see what other options are available. Can you, would you cut back your work hours? When you considered this option six months ago it may not have sounded feasible. Your current situation is much different. Now you *are* a parent, not just thinking about being one. Your priorities may have changed. Could your employer tolerate a change in your job description that would allow you to work fewer hours? What if it were just for six months? This would allow your baby to start solid food and wean to a cup? Or even two months to allow you to regain your stamina?

Can you live on less income? Take a hard look on how you are spending your money. You may be surprised how many corners you can cut to allow yourself to spend more time at home. Every six months or so, I encounter a couple who is struggling with these questions. Although their original plan had been that the new mother would return to work full-time, she finds that separating from her baby is too painful. Although she never dreamed of being a stay-at-home mom, she now realizes that this is how she wants to do it.

Deciding to live on one income is the most difficult part for most young couples. Once they take the leap, they find their lifestyle and spending habits more adaptable than they believed possible. Almost without exception, the couples I know who have decided to get by for a while on one paycheck are pleased with their decision. Please don't interpret these observations as an indictment of the two-income family. For many Americans it is the only option. However, if your return to work has been more chaotic than you expected, take a few days to consider whether you might be able to make ends meet on one income.

Another less drastic option is to reconsider how you and your husband have divided the family-sustaining tasks. Even in families that consider themselves to be egalitarian, women still shoulder the majority of the child-related responsibilities. Of course your husband can't breastfeed his son or daughter, but there are no biological barriers that prevent him from shopping for and preparing meals, doing the laundry, and cleaning the house. Can your husband cut back or reschedule some of his work time so that he can help you get out of the house in the morning or make your return home at the end of the day less chaotic? You may need to think "outside the box" to come up with solutions that will give you enough time and preserve enough of your energy so that you can continue to work and nurse your baby. This is not just *your* problem. It is a *family* problem that requires compromise from every member of the family.

When you have explored all of your options and found that none of them offer practical solutions to your situation, you may be forced to consider weaning. By switching over to formula your body will no longer be expending energy to make milk. The hour or two each day you once spent pumping can be used for other things. If you stop nursing altogether, you can share nighttime feeding responsibilities with a partner. You will no longer be the one who must get up in the middle of the night to feed the baby.

However, before you decide to wean your baby, remember that breastfeeding may not be the only or even the most significant cause of your fatigue and discontentment. Being a parent is an energy-intensive job. Weaning may help you be a bit more efficient, but don't count on the switch to formula to solve all of your problems.

WEANING

You may have been led to believe that weaning your baby is going to be difficult and painful. After watching hundreds of women go through the process, it appears to me that the hardest part is making the decision. Once you commit to the path, the rest of the journey is less difficult, particularly if you have a workable plan and stick to it.

Partial or complete? Do you want or need to completely stop breastfeeding or would you like to retain a few feedings each day? This is not a question you must answer right now because you will be weaning your baby in gradual steps beginning with the feedings that are least important—emotionally, that is—to both of you. You can put the process on hold at any point and reevaluate how the new arrangement fits into your schedule.

I should warn you that your baby or your body may not agree that partial weaning is an option. Your breasts may interpret the decreased demand for milk as a signal to cease production all together. You could try to maintain your supply by frequent pumping, but, if you were weaning to save time and avoid the hassle of pumping, obviously this option doesn't make much sense.

Even if your body maintains its milk production to match your desired feeding schedule, your baby may not be as flexible. Some infants take an all-or-nothing attitude. "Either breastfeed me at every feeding or I won't nurse at all." I'm not sure what prompts some babies to be that way, but it happens. You might end up in a battle of wills and stamina. It is up to you how persistent you want to be. However, I can't guarantee that you are going to win regardless of how stubborn you are.

Which feedings should I drop first? Daytime feedings that correspond to your working hours are the ones to drop first.

The first feeding of the day is probably one you and your baby would like to keep even though it may make getting out of the house in the morning difficult. When you first wake your breasts are full—hopefully after a good long sleep. He is hungry and the first feeding of the day is a wonderful way for you and your baby to say, "Good morning and have a nice day at daycare/work" to each other.

Likewise, the after-work reunion feeding can be a special time for you to reacquaint yourselves and literally reconnect. Unfortunately, your supply may not be up to your baby's demands late in the day. He may willingly accept a supplement bottle of formula after you have nursed for twenty or thirty minutes. On the other hand, your baby may reject you because he wants a full breast or no breast at all. There's really no way to predict what his response will be.

Evening feedings can also have great emotional value. Even if you have been careful not to become your baby's pacifier, nursing may have become an important part of his bedtime ritual, and it is better to hold on to this feeding as long as you can. Remember this doesn't mean feeding your baby until he falls asleep. That is an association we have worked hard to prevent. Nurse him in the living room instead of his bedroom and put on his pajamas after he has nursed. By inserting other components of his bedtime ritual between the nursing and the moment he drifts off to sleep, you will cultivate good sleep habits that will serve you both well in the months and years ahead.

How quickly should I drop feedings? In an emergency you could stop breastfeeding in one day. However, as you might imagine, your baby will find this sudden change upsetting. He is likely to become very cranky and may even refuse a bottle for most of that day. Not to worry, though. Thirst and hunger are powerful motivators. When your baby understands that he can get something wet and sweet out of a bottle, he will eventually take it. (Enlarging the hole in the nipples may help him accept a bottle more readily.) Although he will protest the change in the way he is being fed, your baby will quickly forgive and forget. He will be his happy and contented self again in a couple of days. On the other hand if you have allowed yourself to become a pacifier, this unpleasant transition period can drag on because your baby must not only accept a different method of feeding but must also learn a new way of putting himself to sleep.

Abrupt weaning creates challenges for your body, too. For a few days after you stop nursing, your body will continue to produce significant amounts of milk. Your breasts may become hard, engorged, and painful and may be more vulnerable to mastitis. Traditional suggestions to manage these symptoms include ice packs placed on your breasts and an anti-inflammatory medication such as ibuprofen. Try to resist the temptation to pump your breasts to ease the discomfort because this signals your body to continue making more milk. Another option (if you have time for it) is to continue pumping, but less and less often, over a week or two so that your breasts will gradually adjust to their nonlactating state.

Hopefully, you won't be forced to wean suddenly and can adopt a leisurely schedule. On the first day, substitute the least significant feeding, usually one in the middle of the day, with a bottle of formula. At three months of age you can expect him to take about six ounces, but he could want as many as eight ounces or as few as four. If he is willing to drink, limit the feeding to twenty minutes in length. However, it is more likely that your baby will refuse the bottle and wait impatiently until his next feeding. Resist the temptation to feed him early. Making him wait may not be fun, but your ability to hold out is an important part of making weaning an efficient and humane process. Don't worry about what he's missing nutritionally. Your baby won't become malnourished by skipping one feeding, or even twenty feedings.

Repeat the same schedule on day two. On the third day drop a second feeding. Hold that schedule for a total of two days. Continue to drop a feeding every other day until you arrive at an arrangement that fits your work schedule. If you want to wean more gradually, you could drop a feeding every third or fourth day.

If you are lucky, by the time you have dropped the third feeding your baby will be more than happy to have a bottle instead. It is likely that one bottle may take the place of two or even three feedings, because infants tend to take more at a bottle feeding, and formula generally sits in a stomach longer. However, your baby may decide that he would rather wait until evening and then "power feed" three or four times through the night to make up for the lost daytime nursings. You can decide how you would like to deal with this situation. If fatigue was your primary motivation for weaning, you will probably decide to offer him formula to prevent these extra evening and night feedings. Otherwise you may continue to start each day sleep deprived.

On the other hand, if you were forced to eliminate daytime feedings simply because they didn't fit into your work schedule, you may decide that you are willing to give up some sleep and nurse him several times at night. If you have the stamina, they can provide the two of you with some quality time together.

Regardless of how many feedings you drop, I recommend that you visit the pediatrician for a weight check three or four weeks after you begin weaning. While most babies protest if they are not getting enough to eat, there are some infants who are so content, they stop gaining weight without a whimper. A short trip to the doctor should reassure you that your partial weaning is going well.

Don't waffle. If your baby is being stubborn about weaning, be prepared to be more stubborn. If you give in to his protestations and offer him your breast at a feeding you have decided to eliminate, you will make the next day even more difficult for both of you. When your baby thinks there is even a glimmer of hope that you will nurse him, he will continue to fuss. Once you have decided to wean your baby, carry out the plan. Don't vacillate! To do otherwise amounts to teasing him. Sticking to your plan will make the process go much more quickly and smoothly.

An exception is if your baby gets sick during the weaning process. Then the safe and humane thing to do is to return to your original breastfeeding schedule until the illness has passed. This is particularly true if the illness is gastroenteritis (vomiting and diarrhea). Your breast milk will be much gentler on his system than formula. It will also be easier to keep your baby well hydrated because breast milk has a higher water content than formula. Although illness can interrupt your weaning schedule, the disruption will be temporary. Mutter a bad word or two under your breath and then roll with the punches.

Helping the daycare provider cope. If your baby is one of those stubborn little buggers who initially refuses to take a bottle, your daycare provider may need some support to help her ride out those first few rocky days. Experienced and unflappable daycare providers will have seen it all before and will be the ones comforting you. If your daycare provider has never dealt with a weaning baby, be quick to reassure her that your baby will not starve. Warn her before you begin the process so that she can prepare herself for a fussy day or two. You might even suggest that she add another staff person (and offer to pay for their time!) to help her deal with the chaos created by your stubborn baby. Offer to pay extra because she (and not you) is the one who must endure your baby's fussiness.

A few more bumps in the road. Introducing formula to your baby may be associated with other unanticipated problems. The most common reaction is constipation. Breast milk is a natural laxative, and although nursing babies may have infrequent bowel movements, they are invariably loose. The addition of even small amounts of formula to your baby's diet may make his stools firm and difficult to pass. This change may be a minor nuisance while your baby learns that he will have to use his abdominal muscles to have a bowel movement.

Unfortunately, some infants have more troublesome constipation. Before you begin switching formulas in an attempt to help, wait a few days. Often things will improve with time. A glycerin suppository once a day for a few days may be all that is necessary to help your baby over the transition. If your baby needs suppositories on a regular basis, it is time to talk to your pediatrician about changing formulas. She may suggest that you try first a little diluted apple, white grape, or prune juice. Keep in mind that making a change in your child's diet may not noticeably affect your child's bowel movement for several days. Occasionally, I encounter families frustrated by their failure to find a dietary remedy for their child's constipation or a formula that will agree with their baby's digestive system. Often the solution lies in a juice or formula that had been previously discarded after a trial that had lasted only a day or two. Remember that some infants get gassy and crampy when they are offered too much juice or juice that isn't sufficiently diluted. This discomfort may be misinterpreted as constipation. Move slowly and patiently as you make changes.

Constipation is only one symptom of formula intolerance. Most babies spit up more when they are fed formula, but a few babies will actually regurgitate less when they are weaned off of breast milk because the thicker formula is less likely to slosh back up. As long your baby is comfortable and gaining weight, spitting up is seldom justification for a new formula. On the other hand, projectile vomiting, poor weight gain, and apparent abdominal pain can be symptoms of formula intolerance. Explosive diarrhea and gassiness may also indicate a formula change is in order.

For years physicians have suggested a soy-based formula for babies troubled by traditional cow's-milk formulas. Unfortunately, many infants seem to be more constipated with soy formula. If constipation is your child's primary problem I suggest that you first try other cow's-milk formulas, particularly a lactose-free one. While other parents may be quick to offer well-meaning advice, recognize that your baby's digestive system may not respond in the same way as another child's. You will probably have to do some experimenting on your own.

It may surprise you to read that there is little, if any, evidence that iron-fortified formulas are more likely to cause constipation. In fact, I recommend them. There are several "elemental" formulas that can be used when standard formulas don't seem to be the answer. However, I urge you to consult your pediatrician in your search for a formula that agrees with your baby.

True formula "allergy," as opposed to "intolerance," is unusual. However, if your baby develops hives or turns red the first time you offer him formula, contact your pediatrician promptly. These are signs of a potentially significant allergy. Do not offer any more formula without her guidance. Other rashes are usually less important, and in my experience are generally not related to formula changes.

Though there may be some evidence that children who are breastfed have fewer ear infections, don't feel guilty if your baby gets more colds and ear infections after you wean him. Close contact with his germ-laden daycare mates is by far the more likely cause.

22

THE REST OF THE STORY (MONTHS FOUR THROUGH TWELVE)

Even though you had always planned to wean your baby when he was three months old, you may have found breastfeeding easier and more fun than you had imagined. Now you would like to nurse for a another few months or even longer. I hope this change in plan is to some extent the result of the *Maternity Leave Breastfeeding Plan*'s emphasis on fatigue prevention, but whatever the reason, your baby and I are pleased that you will be continuing for a while longer. You have already cleared the biggest hurdles, but challenges remain. This chapter will guide you through the next nine months—until your child's first birthday.

Making a new and longer plan. You may simply want to take one week at a time and continue to nurse only as long as you have the time and energy. Way back in Chapter 7, I told you that when you no longer felt fulfilled by breastfeeding it was time to stop and I cautioned you not to feel guilty about your decision. It is impossible to predict what stresses life will bring you in the next six months. Your job may become more demanding or a family member's illness may force you to take on the role of part-time caregiver for that person, for example. Your plan to nurse your baby until he wants to stop may have to be scaled back to accommodate unforeseen changes in your life.

Though the future is unpredictable, you may feel more comfortable if you have a loosely drawn schedule of what to expect from breastfeeding for the next six months. Many families I see in my practice offer solid foods when their baby is four months old and introduce a cup at five months of age. *If* he accepts the solids eagerly and *if* he becomes skillful with the cup, the baby can be weaned from the breast and bottle feedings by the time he is nine months old and the hassle with bottles is avoided. The next two sections will tell you how to begin the gradual transition from a diet that is an all-liquid diet to one that is similar to yours. Unfortunately, some babies would rather advance their diet at a more leisurely pace, and there isn't much you can or should do to rush the process.

Adding solids. For the first ten years I was in practice I encouraged parents to limit their babies to breast milk or formula for the first six months. Like most pediatricians at that time, I believed the introduction of solid food during the first half year was not only unnecessary but that it exposed babies to a significantly increased risk of allergy and gastrointestinal injury. It was a mighty struggle. We pitted ourselves against grandmothers, aunts, and next-door neighbors who were advising parents to give their young infants baby food to help grow faster and sleep through the night. Some parents followed my suggestions and waited, but most caved in under the heavy pressure from friends and family and began giving their babies cereal at four months of age or even earlier. A few of these "disobedient" parents sheepishly volunteered to me the "error" of their ways, but most would fess up only if I quizzed them repeatedly.

Fortunately, I eventually wised up and now realize that while most infants do not require solid food until they are six months old, or in some cases even eight or nine months old, there's nothing wrong with starting babies on cereal at four months. While there can be complications associated with the introduction of solids, they are usually relatively minor and occur infrequently. In fact beginning solids as early as four months can be an important factor in helping some mothers achieve their goal of continuing to breastfeed their babies when they return to work. I have also encountered a few babies who are growing so quickly that by time they are four months old they have outstripped their mother's milk production. These tigers need the extra calories that solid foods provide. These are usually very large babies or ones whose mothers have become fatigued.

Before we launch into the specifics of adding solids, let me caution you that if you or your husband have a family history of allergies, asthma, or eczema, ignore my suggestions about broadening your baby's diet at four months. While there is only spotty evidence that waiting another few months will decrease the risk of your child developing these conditions, it's prudent to keep him on breast milk alone for the first six months if you can.

Traditionally the first solid food offered to babies is rice cereal. It is easy to digest and baby food manufacturers fortify it with iron, the first nutritional element that your baby may need in excess of that found in your breast milk. Mix just a tablespoon or two of the dry cereal with your breast milk for the first feeding. If you don't have breast milk to spare, you can use water. Eventually diluting with apple juice or formula would be acceptable, but initially you want to be careful to *introduce only one new food at a time*. This concept is important, so I will remind you about it again. The mixture should be very watery for the first few feedings and given on a spoon. With very rare exceptions, if a baby is too small or immature to be fed with a spoon, he is too young for solid food.

The first week or two offer just one rice cereal feeding a day. Usually morning or late afternoon works best, but if your baby seems extra hungry at lunchtime, that would be fine. Don't make this solid feeding a bedtime snack. We want to preserve his good sleeping habits and this means keeping solid foods out of his bedtime ritual. Despite what you have heard, most babies will not sleep better if you load them up with solids before they go to bed for the night.

Keep the volumes small for the first week, just a few teaspoonfuls at the most. Even if your baby is eager for his cereal from his first taste, resist the temptation to stuff him. His digestive tract needs some time to adjust, and his eyes may be bigger than his stomach. In a few weeks you can let him eat until his body language tells you that he has had enough. Whenever you introduce any new food, keep the amounts modest for the first few feedings.

After a week you can begin to offer him cereal twice a day if he is interested. These offerings should come *after* nursings. Breast milk should remain his primary nutrition for the next two or three months. After that your baby will tell you when he prefers to start his feedings with solids and will treat your milk more as a beverage.

If your baby acts as though you are trying to poison him when you approach him with a spoon, relax. We have plenty of time. This isn't a race. However, don't quit, just keep offering day after day. If the attempts at solids become an ugly scene, back off for a week or two and then try again. Try mixing the cereal with juice or pureed fruit, but don't write your baby off as a picky eater before he is six months old. Some finicky eaters are unwittingly conditioned to stay that way because their parents give up on offering new foods too quickly. It may take up to fifteen or twenty attempts before you succeed. I am not suggesting that you force-feed your baby. I am merely urging you to be persistent. (A more in-depth discussion of managing finicky eaters can be found in my first book, *Coping with a Picky Eater*, Simon & Schuster, 1998.)

It is extremely unlikely that your baby will have an allergic reaction to rice cereal, or to any of the other standard baby foods, for that matter. However, you should be alert for rashes, particularly hives or generalized redness and particularly around his mouth or bottom. More than his usual spitting up or outright vomiting are other signs of a food intolerance or allergy.

Expect a change in bowel movements as you introduce new foods. You are changing what goes in so you shouldn't be surprised that something different comes out. The most common change would be toward a harder, more formed bowel movement. This is particularly true of bananas and for that reason I suggest you offer them after other fruits. Explosive watery bowel movements and/or gassy behavior is a warning to avoid the offending food for awhile before trying it again.

A complete discussion of baby foods is beyond the scope of this book, but I will put in my two cents worth about a couple of issues. First, there are many appropriate ways to introduce solids—and very few wrong ones. As long as you don't offer more than one new food at a time you will usually be able to detect when your child is allergic or intolerant. The process is made easier if you include the new food in meals for three or four days in a row to gain consistent experience with it. Remember to introduce just one new food at a time.

The notion that if you introduce fruits before vegetables your child will develop a sweet tooth and never enjoy vegetables is bunk. Particularly if you are giving your baby cereal for breakfast, fruit is just a more natural companion. I suggest that you add fruits after your child has checked out on rice cereal. The truth is it really doesn't make any difference.

When your child is ready to advance to a third food category—for example, adding vegetables after rice cereal and fruit—it's time to add a third solid meal. Remember there is no rush. Your child has an entire lifetime to eat solid food.

Introducing a cup. Although you may not plan on weaning your baby for another six or eight months, the transition will go more smoothly if you gradually introduce him to a cup at about five months of age. Many parents inadvertently begin the process as early as four months, when they yield to their babies' curiosity and allow them a sip of iced tea or soft drink out of their own glasses.

Begin by using a standard plastic or sturdy glass cup or tumbler. Training cups with spouts confuse young infants because they try to suck on the spout and become frustrated when they discover it doesn't work like a nipple. On the other hand, they will eagerly hook their gums over the open rim of a cup or glass as you gradually tip it up for them. Have a face cloth or paper towel on hand because the first few times most of the contents will run down their chin as they try to lap it up like a cat or dog. With time they will become more skillful, and after several months they will be able hold a training cup themselves. Obviously at that point the addition of a lid that discourages massive spills would be a good idea. My favorite cup is one with a recessed cover with two holes which allow a swallow of liquid to be released when tipped up, but won't empty when inverted accidentally, or otherwise.

You can start with water, but I have found that the slightly sweet taste of diluted apple or white grape juice helps interest babies in the cup. Don't waste your money on "baby" juices. Pasteurized "adult" juice diluted with four or five parts of water to one part juice is all you need. Schedule these messy little training sessions midway between feedings. Eventually these will become your baby's midmorning and midafternoon snack times. If he coughs and sputters or doesn't like the concept, back off and come back to it a week or two later. It won't be too long before your baby really gets into the fun (and mess) of drinking from a cup.

Once he is reasonably accomplished, his newfound drinking skill will make separations of a few hours that much easier. While we can't expect your baby to keep himself well nourished for days with only a cup, he will be able to quench his thirst and stay contented until you get home. By the time he is nine months old it is very possible that he will be able to grow and thrive on a combination of baby food and table food and what he can drink from a cup (formula or whole milk). Hundreds of patients have achieved this level of nutritional sophistication well before their first birthdays and in doing so have allowed their mothers to stop breastfeeding. Unfortunately, I can't guarantee that your baby will become this motivated or skillful by the time he is nine months old, but by introducing a cup at four or five months of age you will lay a foundation that he can build on when he is ready.

Unless your pediatrician has suggested it as a treatment for constipation, don't give your baby juice in a bottle. Drinking juice from a bottle can become a nasty habit that can be very difficult to break. Too much juice can interfere with your baby's natural appetite, give him diarrhea, and contribute to tooth decay. Make a rule now that the only way your baby will get juice is from a cup. It will head off a host of problems before they can get started.

The cutting edge (what to do when your baby bites you). Most babies don't cut teeth until they are entering their second six months. However, teeth can erupt at any time. Equipped with these sharp little weapons your baby may begin to bite or chew on your nipple. When this happens, go with your first instinct. Yelp loudly and stop the feeding. This will usually alert your baby that he has made a mistake and hopefully discourage him from biting you again.

Unfortunately, many mothers suffer in silence and their babies never get the message that they are inflicting pain. Your baby doesn't know he is hurting you unless you tell him in a way that he can understand. This means that if your baby is beginning to bite, your response should be swift, loud, and forceful. Don't worry if your cry leads to tears on his part. His desire to nurse will bring him back to your breast, but hopefully he will think twice rather than bite you again.

Should I continue to nurse when I'm sick? The answer to this question is almost always yes. There are very few illnesses that are passed through breast milk alone. Most germs that cause child-hood illnesses are spread hand-to-mouth or float in the air. Upper respiratory infections (colds) and gastroenteritis (stomach flu) are best prevented by good hand-washing habits. Masks and gloves won't make a difference.

The few exceptions to this general rule include serious viral infections such as HIV (the virus that causes AIDS) and certain forms of hepatitis. When in doubt, call your pediatrician for advice. Most of the time she will tell you that the advantages of breastfeeding outweigh any minimal risk that you will make your baby sick by nursing when you are ill.

You must also consider your own health when deciding whether it is wise to continue nursing when you are sick. Breastfeeding is a nutritional and fluid drain on you. It may be wise to skip a feeding or two so that you can get some rest and restore your body fluids. This is particularly true if you have had vomiting and/or diarrhea. If you stop nursing altogether for more than a day, you may find it difficult to rebuild your milk production. Instead try short, occasional pumping sessions to remind your body that it has a job to do when you are feeling better. These kinds of decisions should be made in consultation with your own physician and the pediatrician. The issue of what medications you can safely take is discussed in Appendix III.

Long separations. If you decide to breastfeed for more than three months, you may encounter a situation that requires you to be away from your baby for more than twelve hours—a two-day business trip or a romantic getaway weekend, for instance.

I don't need to warn you that leaving your baby for more than a day is going to be an emotional challenge. In fact, I will be surprised if your husband is able to convince you to sneak away for at least another year. If you are able to overcome your natural resistance to leave your baby behind, consider what effect the separation will have on breastfeeding.

A combination of the stress of traveling and the lack of natural stimulation to your breasts may send your milk production into a downward spiral from which it may never recover. If you have always been a bountiful producer, this is unlikely, but I don't know of any way to guarantee you that it won't happen. Of course you will improve your chances of keeping your milk supply up by bringing your pump along with you. To do otherwise would certainly mark the end of your nursing career.

I must warn you that your baby will have something to say about what happens when you return from your trip. Most babies will be so eager to see their mothers again that they will forgive and forget and nurse as often as it takes to rebuild your milk supply. However, you may have one of those babies who holds a grudge and refuses to nurse when you return. The solution lies in your ability to be more stubborn than your baby. Don't offer him any other source of nutrition or fluid until he finally accepts that you are still the source from which all good things flow. Most healthy babies can safely fast for twelve hours, but it usually doesn't take this long for them to realize that they should be nursing. You may want to check with your pediatrician to see if she agrees that this guideline applies to your baby.

If your supply has dipped dramatically while you were away, you may not be able to play this waiting game because your baby will receive little reward when he returns to your breast. But, continue to pump in hopes that your milk will return in force. Even if managed properly, an extended separation of even one day or two may signal the end to nursing.

Another solution is to bring your baby along with you. I know several mothers who have been able to arrange accommodations and business meeting schedules around nursing and caring for their baby. However, many babies will find the traveling so tiring and sleeping in strange places so unnerving that it hardly seems worth the effort. Hopefully, by the time your first business trip appears on your schedule you will understand your baby well enough to predict how he would tolerate being your traveling companion.

Weaning II. In the last chapter I described several approaches to weaning your baby when he was still dependent on liquid nutrition. It is time to revisit the issue now that he has begun taking solid food. First, remember that it is unlikely that your infant will be able to sustain adequate growth without a substantial contribution from your breast or bottles of formula until he is at least eight or nine months of age. He just won't be skillful enough with a cup nor will he be eating enough solid food before then. In other words, if you plan to wean your baby before he is nine months of age, you should wean him to a bottle.

If he can drink three or four ounces of formula or whole milk from a cup three or four times a day, you can consider weaning him without making a detour through a bottle stage. Although this advice runs counter to the nutritional party line, I think it is perfectly all right to wean your baby to whole milk before he is a year of age as long as it is being given to him in a cup. I believe that as long as your child is drinking from a bottle that it should contain formula or breast milk. The reason for this is that while the liquid he drinks from a cup is a relatively small portion of his diet, bottles may contain a much larger volume of liquid and can add up to a significant percentage of his daily nutrition. Cow's milk in large volumes may displace more important nutritional elements from your baby's diet.

If your baby initiates the weaning process, your job is easy. By the time he is seven months of age he may have whittled down his nursing (or bottles) to three a day. As long as his pediatrician is happy with his growth, don't worry. It may take him another few months to drop these last three feedings, but by the time he is eight or nine months old he will be able to fly on his own.

On the other hand, some babies are really into sucking and will not show any inclination to drop feedings unless you initiate the change. As I discussed in previous chapters, you can and should wean your baby whenever you feel the time is right. This can be a hard decision. You enjoy these special times together, but the demands of your job and other obligations may be making it increasingly difficult to fit nursing into your schedule. Of course it is easier when it is his idea, but you won't create any deep emotional scars as long as you move at a slow and steady pace. The thing to avoid is waffling. Flip-flopping back and forth from day to day will make weaning much harder on both of you. Your baby is counting on your leadership. He will find it very unsettling if you cut back from four to three nursings, then two days later go back to four. Don't make the process any more difficult than it needs to be by sending your baby mixed messages. You've already laid the groundwork for the process in carefully avoiding becoming his pacifier.

Usually the best feeding to drop first is the midday feeding because your baby has the least emotional and nutritional investment in it. This strategy will also fit nicely into your work schedule if you'll be working from nine till five. You may discover that both you and your baby want to retain a nursing at the beginning and the end of the day for many more months. Even after they have lost most of their nutritional significance, these feedings will continue to give you both a quiet time to renew physical closeness.

Unless you are faced with an emergency that requires an abrupt and complete cessation, I suggest you wait at least three or four days before you drop the next feeding. This will give both of your bodies—and your child's expectations—time to adjust. Offer him frequent opportunities to drink from a cup or bottle as you continue the weaning process.

Even if you take things slowly, your baby may protest and make it very clear what he is missing. Resist reinstituting feedings that you have dropped! Slow down the weaning process if you like, but don't relinquish any ground you have struggled to gain. On the other hand, if your child becomes ill, particularly if it is a gastrointestinal upset, don't hesitate to return some or all of the feedings you have dropped. It may help him feel better, both physically and emotionally. Chalk it up to bad luck and resume your plan when he is healthy again.

Extended nursing. Although when you bought this book you had absolutely no intention of continuing to nurse when your maternity leave was over, things change. Nursing has been more fun than you ever expected and less of a hassle. Your child may still enjoy sitting in your lap a couple of times a day to breastfeed even though he is a toddler. It just sort of happened.

Don't worry about it, just enjoy the experience. You will encounter people who find what you are doing unsettling and even distasteful, but as long as nursing is something that both of you want to do, it's fine. There is nothing biologically or psychologically wrong with nursing a two or three year old. To be honest, most of the women I know who are still nursing toddlers have allowed themselves to become pacifiers, and I wonder if they had avoided this trap whether they would still want to breastfeed. On the other hand, I know plenty of mothers whose children can sleep independently and have enjoyed extended nursing.

If you become pregnant again, you will want to rethink your continued nursing and to discuss this with your obstetrician. Breastfeeding does create a nutritional drag on your body and can stimulate uterine contractions, which can threaten the pregnancy. I suspect that your obstetrician will encourage you to wean your toddler.

23

NURSING YOUR SECOND CHILD

Breastfeeding your first child may not have been as positive an experience as you had hoped. You may have limped through months or even a year feeling that the sacrifice was worth it because your child's health was at stake. Nevertheless you felt trapped and exhausted by nursing. Possibly you ended up as your child's pacifier and have promised yourself that it's not going to happen again. Or perhaps your first baby thrived on your breast milk, but you stopped nursing after a few months because breast-feeding or the combination of work and breastfeeding was taking too much out of you. You would like to try again, but this time make a little more time for yourself and the rest of your family. There is a better way and this book can help.

On the other hand you may be having your second (or third) child, but this is your first attempt at nursing. You may have been too young, too busy, or perhaps you simply lacked the confidence to breastfeed. You may have since learned more about the benefits of breastfeeding and would like to give your next child some hope of preventing the ear infections that plagued your first child. You may regret shying away from the challenge the first time and now would like to give it your best shot.

Whatever your history, you find yourself in the position of wanting to nurse a new baby with another child in the house. Depending on the age of the older sibling, you will encounter a variety of challenges that a first-time parent won't.

If you sense that your school-age child is uncomfortable with your breastfeeding, talk to him about the reasons why you have chosen to nurse and ask him to tell you what he is feeling. You may have to breastfeed discreetly at home as though you were out in public. It may be not what you had planned, but hopefully the older child will become more comfortable with the concept as the weeks pass. Remember, you are all part of a family, and sympathy for the ambivalence of your preadolescent will allow you and the new baby to enjoy nursing and still maintain harmony at home.

If your first child is a toddler or preschooler (aged eighteen months to five years), breastfeeding may signal the first major battle in that perennial war known as sibling rivalry. It is hard enough for your first child to share your attention with anyone else, but when you are giving your breast to the new baby, a breast that he once considered his own, don't be surprised if the older-child response is less than positive. Tantrums and mischievous behavior are likely to erupt, especially just as you sit down to feed the baby.

While most parents expect sibling rivalry to manifest itself as physical attacks directed at the younger child, it is much more likely that you will be the target of physical and verbal abuse. Older children aren't stupid; they know the baby didn't ask to come into the world. They know that you and your husband, not the baby, are the bad guys. It was you who decided to bring this stranger into the house and disrupt what had been a peaceful family in which everyone had their space and everyone got enough attention. Now, thanks to you, your older child's life has suddenly been turned upside down. You are the one who will pay for it.

Ads in baby magazines often picture beautifully coifed young mothers, breastfeeding their babies in the quiet solitude of a tastefully decorated nursery. You can almost hear the harp playing in the background. Achieving this idyllic atmosphere is difficult enough when it is just you and your newborn; it is downright impossible if you have another young child in the house. A more realistic picture would show a disheveled woman sitting on a couch trying to keep her toddler from poking a Lego block in the baby's ear, with piles of children's books and toys littering the floor at her feet. Actually that picture is a bit optimistic—at least the toddler is within arm's reach. More likely he will be running off to some distant corner of the house looking for mischief.

It is surprising that any mothers with more than one child can relax enough to make milk, let alone find the time to get it to the baby. Toddlers have an uncanny instinct for timing and will often want an escort to the bathroom just as you are settling down on the couch to nurse a younger brother or sister. Disruptive behavior may go beyond the usual random violence one can expect from a two or three year old. Clearly there are situations when an action is intended to get your attention, or at least divert it from his rival. Whether intentional or not, you can count on most toddlers to make your attempts at nursing far from the quiet bonding sessions that you remember from the first time around.

You have two challenges. One is logistical. You must somehow figure out how to feed one more mouth and clean one more bottom in the same twenty-four hours you once had to care for a single child. The other challenge is creating an illusion that will convince your first child that nothing has changed and he is getting just as much attention as before his new baby brother or sister was born.

The logistical challenge can be met with a combination of planning and reprioritization. You will need an extra set of hands for the first month or two, until the new baby is nursing less often and the older child has come to accept the inevitability of the intruder sticking around. Hopefully your husband can take some time off from work to help entertain the older child and get at least some of the chores done. Grandparents, aunts, uncles, and family friends can also be enlisted as support personnel.

Helpers should be prepared to perform a wide variety of functions. In the morning the older child may want Grandma's undivided attention, but by afternoon he has grown tired of this diversion and wants you. At that point your helper must shift gears and take over the less enjoyable tasks of changing the baby, doing the laundry, and fixing supper. Don't feel bad about this turn of events—we're not calling them helpers for nothing! The next day the pattern may be reversed. The more skillful you are at reading your older child's emotional needs, and the more flexible that you and your helpers can be, the easier the transition from only child to sibling will be.

Everyone in the family should be aware of the fragile emotional state of the older child. The sensitive adult will be careful to not pay too much attention to the new baby. Interest in the newborn should be funneled through the sibling. "Robbie, you look so much bigger than the baby. Can we go over and look at her together?" is an example of an approach that will help defuse some of the sibling tension.

Whether you have a helper or not, you will need to reprioritize if you are going to succeed in nursing and keeping chaos at bay. Don't worry if the dust piles up. Don't worry if the menus lean more toward take-out and frozen dinners. You will get things back on a more even keel in a few weeks. No one is going to starve to death or die from multiplying dust bunnies while you are taking the time to get your nursing off to a good start.

At the same time you are trying to solve the logistical challenges, you must also engage in a bit of magical deception. To give the older child time to adjust to his new role, you must create the illusion that although there is another person in the house, everything will be just the way it was before the baby was born. Obviously this deception is going to be less than perfect, but you will be rewarded for your efforts.

First, try to keep intact the older child's daily schedule. The ultimate plan may be for big brother to continue his established daycare schedule, but you must be sensitive to his perception of the plan. If he feels as though he is being shunted off and is missing out on the real fun of being around the new baby, then you will want to delay his return to daycare for a few weeks. Simple things like preserving lunch and snack times and walks to the playground can create a sense of stability that will help the big brother or sister feel more comfortable with sibship. Of course this may mean juggling the new baby's nursing schedule by a few minutes here and there, but everyone has to give a little, including the baby.

Don't forget that for the first month or two of life your new baby should be sleeping most of the time and feeding the rest. Take advantage of this initial period of relative inactivity. The new baby needs to nurse for a half hour every few hours, but the rest of the day she should be in her room, in her bed, out of sight. Your first child was a novelty, a new toy to play with. You felt that he needed to be talked to and played with every waking hour. He really didn't, but you did it anyway because it was fun and you had the time. Your curiosity and inexperience probably kept him awake when he should have been asleep. Things have changed dramatically. You don't have the time, and, besides, for the first two months all you really need to do is feed your new baby and then put her right down to bed. For your older child this means that the new baby is "out of sight and out of mind." At least some of the day things are back to the way they were before the intruder arrived.

Take advantage of this time and spend it with the older brother or sister. Don't waste it on housework or cooking meals. In a couple of months the baby is going to be demanding and deserving more attention. You will no longer be able to put her down right after a feeding. She will be up for at least half an hour or more. Hopefully by that time the older sibling will have become more accustomed to sharing the limelight.

The baby will have to be nursed frequently in the first few weeks, and you will have to develop a strategy for keeping your older child amused while you are breastfeeding. Ideally, the three of you can all sit on the couch, and you and the older child can read a story together or watch a video. Unfortunately, many young children just don't have the patience to stay seated for the entire twenty or thirty minutes it may take to nurse the baby no matter how interesting you try to make it. They will want to get up and run around a little. One solution is to nurse in a space that you can easily secure. This may mean adding latches and setting up gates or, during warmer weather, nursing in a fenced-in backyard. "Child proof" (an oxymoron if there ever was one) the area so that you can allow the child to roam freely.

If your older child's behavior becomes disruptive, you may have to banish him to his room until the nursing session is over. Many parents have trouble with the concept of latching their child in his room as a disciplinary measure, but often it is the only safe solution to a difficult situation. The child will *not* come to hate his room, though it is likely that he will pitch quite a fuss as you are putting him in there. This confrontation may upset you and make it difficult for you to relax enough to nurse. Hopefully after a few days, the older sibling will learn that if he behaves, he will be able to stay with you while you nurse or accept the fact that he is better off playing in his room while the baby feeds.

In some families an older child's needs for attention make it impossible for his mother to nurse successfully or enjoyably. Weaning may be the only solution, but there are two other strategies to consider first. One is to hire a babysitter to come into your home and amuse big brother or sister during the feedings. Obviously, this is an expensive option, particularly if it takes several months for the older sibling to adjust. On the other hand if nursing is something that you enjoy and want to continue, it may be worth the expense.

A second option often evolves naturally. The baby may begin to realize that the evening and night feedings are much more relaxed because the disruptive older sibling has gone to bed. She may begin to refuse the hectic daytime feedings and wake to feed more often at night. If your baby chooses this option, you will need to ask yourself if you have the stamina to be up every few hours at night to breastfeed and still have the energy to chase a two year old during the day. These preferential night feedings may continue for several months longer than with your first child, and so your hopes of the baby sleeping through the night may need to be put on hold.

Your decision to continue nursing in the face of a challenging two or three year old and the specter of going back to work is all your own. As you know I am not in favor of martyrdom. Remember you are in the business of building a family comprised of healthy and happy individuals, which includes yourself. To be a good mother, a supportive spouse, and an effective worker, you must be rested and have a piece of yourself left over at the end of the day. If nursing and chasing a toddler make that impossible, the better part of valor may be to wean the baby, either partially or completely. Breastfeeding is very important, but not worth you being a miserable and exhausted parent.

24

In Defense of Realism

As I finished the last draft of *The Maternity Leave Breastfeeding Plan* I began preparing myself for the criticism that I knew might come. I predicted that some breastfeeding advocates might label me a pessimist and accuse me of setting back breastfeeding in this country by twenty years.

I could hear their argument: Encouraging women to breastfeed for "only" three months and telling them that they should wean their babies when they no longer enjoyed nursing would lead to fewer and fewer breastfed babies. If a three-month nursing career was adopted as the unofficial standard, I could be blamed for weakening our position with the government and business leaders who must take action if longer maternity leaves are to become a reality.

My response to those criticisms will be that the numbers—the hundreds of women who have brought their children to my office—speak for themselves. Unrealistic nursing goals do not encourage more women to nurse longer. We have nothing to lose by taking a more realistic approach to breastfeeding that acknowledges the challenges faced by working women in North America.

Our current strategy of asking women to nurse for longer periods of time has actually discouraged some of them from starting and has made countless others feel guilty when they fail to meet our expectations. I am confident that as more women like yourself discover that three months of breastfeeding is a legitimate and admirable goal, we will find that more women *begin* nursing. And, as more women learn how to avoid becoming their babies' pacifiers, they will nurse longer because they are enjoying it more.

I also anticipate that some critics will claim that I have underestimated the strength and determination of women. Nothing could be further from the truth. I was raised in a family in which my mother was the one with the driver's license, the college degree, and the mechanical skills to fix my broken toys and bicycles. Although my father has always been a kind and caring parent, my mother was the take-charge, get-it-done person. She worked outside the home long before it became the norm and was a feared and respected negotiator among the business community in our hometown. My wife has also worked outside the home and breastfed our three children. She has overcome a variety of orthopedic problems and bicycled four thousand miles across the country.

These two remarkable women and scores of others have convinced me that women are at least as capable of accepting and mastering life's challenges as men. However, breastfeeding is *not* a competitive sport. While some women can continue to nurse when they return to work, this does not mean that every woman is expected to turn herself into a sleep-deprived zombie to meet unrealistic expectations.

The time has come to inject common sense and realism into our approach to breastfeeding.

Appendix 1.

Burping Your Baby

Most of the gas in your baby's digestive tract is air he has swallowed during feedings, and he is the one who is ultimately responsible for getting it back out by burping. You are merely an enabler in the process. In three or four months he will have mastered the skill of burping by himself.

In Chapter 17 I cautioned you to burp your baby early in the feeding, before the air he has swallowed has had a chance to move farther downstream. Once the gas has moved into his intestines, it simply can't be released with a burp. Remember that your baby is the one doing the burping. If he falls into a deep sleep, he probably won't be able to do the job.

Begin with your baby sitting on your lap, facing either right or left, whichever is most comfortable for you. Support his chin with the thumb and first fingers of one hand, so that his head can't flop forward. This will straighten his esophagus and allow the air a clear passage for its final few inches before it comes out his mouth. If your hand is big enough, the pinky finger of that hand can press *gently* under his ribs. This adds a little to the abdominal pressure he will create by himself. Your other hand should be supporting his back.

Next allow your baby to slowly rock onto his back. Initially, he may balk at this change in position. All babies are afraid of falling, and some get very nervous until they become confident that you will support them. Keep him on his back for a slow count of five.

Then slowly tip him back to his original sitting position but bent slightly forward at the waist, which is folded over the pinky you have tucked under his ribs. With your other hand firmly rub his back in a circular motion. This is likely to encourage your baby to contract his back muscles and sit more upright, which may help the gas out.

Alternate this circular rubbing with the traditional patting between his shoulder blades. After he has been sitting for a slow count of ten, lay him back down. Repeat the cycle several times. If he hasn't burped after three or four minutes, allow your baby to return to your breast. Dragging out the process will only exhaust your baby and make him more cranky.

The gas bubbles are most likely to come up as your baby goes from lying to sitting. Parents who prefer burping with the over-the-shoulder technique often find that the burps come as they are transferring their baby from their lap to their shoulder. This is really the same motion that I am suggesting, but keeping it all on your lap makes cleanup easier if your baby spits up.

This burping technique was taught to me by an experienced nursery nurse while I was a medical student. Over the years, it has proven the most effective technique, and we've seen and tried a lot. However, you and your baby must discover the system that works best for you. Remember, whatever technique you use, initiate it early in the feeding and don't drag it out too long.

Appendix 2.

What Medications Can I Take While I Am Nursing?

As with any breastfeeding issue there is as much myth and confusion surrounding this question as any breastfeeding issue. On the one hand, the answer is very simple. Most of the medications that your doctor might prescribe for you are safe to take while you are nursing. However, before you consider taking any medication, you should thoroughly investigate and consider its risks and benefits to both you and your baby.

Do you really need the medication? We are a drug-seeking society. We prefer quick and easy answers to our problems; if we can pull one off the shelf in the form of a pill, all the better. I trust that during your pregnancy the fear of taking something that might harm your unborn baby prompted you to reconsider your usual medication-taking practices. Most women find that they can weather colds and viral illnesses without the over-the-counter drugs they were accustomed to taking before pregnancy.

Most physicians will tell you that over-the-counter medications are often ineffective and frequently have at least as many side effects as benefits. You will get over your cold or stomach flu just as quickly whether you take medication or not. Plenty of fluids and a box of tissues will see you through most colds. If you feel you must take something for nasal stuffiness, consider a nasal spray rather than an oral medication. Most nursing babies can tolerate breast milk that has been tainted with antihistamines or

Sudafed, but some will become drowsy or agitated when exposed to common cold-medication ingredients. Ask your physician to help you pick an over-the-counter medication and avoid combinations that may contain far more ingredients than you need. The bottom line is that you should not take any over-the-counter or prescription medication without the approval of your physician.

If your physician prescribes a medication, make sure that you discuss with her the necessity of the medication and alternatives. Would physical therapy, or a dietary change, or simply watchful waiting be just as effective? There's no reason to suffer if you need medication. You must be comfortable if you are going to be a good mother. However, make sure that you have discussed alternative chemical-free therapies with your physician.

Remind your physician that you are breastfeeding. If your obstetrician is also your primary care provider, she will probably be aware that you are nursing. However, make no assumptions! Before you walk out of the office or hang up the phone, ask, "Doctor, will this medication be safe to take while I am breastfeeding?" If you sense any hesitancy in her voice, ask her to double-check and/or get a second opinion.

Unfortunately, there has been very little research done on the safety of taking medication while breastfeeding. This means that your doctor will have very few resources to consult. Literature from the manufacturers will more than likely read, "No data is available about *medication x* and breast milk." Or, she may discover a reference that says, "Two cases have been reported in which nursing mothers took *medication x* while they were nursing. The researchers could detect no ill effects in the infants."

You can imagine that this will put your physician in a difficult position. Should she prescribe a medication for you based on two successful experiences? That really isn't very many.

Is there a safer medication? If there is only scanty information on the medication that you have been prescribed, can your physician find a safer alternative? She may have to do some more reading and a bit of calling around to find the answer. If she is not an obstetrician or pediatrician, suggest that she call one of these specialists who usually have more experience with medication and breastfeeding. I often field calls like these.

Most of the medications you are prescribed are safe. This includes most antibiotics and pain medications, which are the two most common kinds of medicines prescribed after childbirth. Some babies will become a bit drowsy when their mothers are taking strong pain medications, and yeast infections in the form of thrush and diaper rash are more likely to occur when babies are exposed to antibiotics. However, these are generally minor issues and should not prevent you from taking the medication that has been prescribed.

The antidepressants, particularly those referred to as SSRIs (Paxil, Prozac, and Zoloft are the most frequently prescribed), have been used safely by thousands of nursing mothers. However, you should discuss your treatment options with your doctor before restarting any medication while you are nursing.

The list of medications that we know are unsafe for nursing mothers is actually rather short. Lithium, which is used to treat depression, is one. Most of the others are chemotherapy agents used for cancer treatment. Some radioactive tracers that are used in certain diagnostic scans can also be a problem.

Unacceptable medications. If you must take a medication that is incompatible with breastfeeding, ask if the treatment or the diagnostic scan can be delayed so that you can have a few more weeks of nursing. Obviously you should not put your own health at risk simply to continue breastfeeding.

If your treatment will last for just a week or two, you may want to pump and discard your milk until the last traces of medication have left your body. Then you can safely return to nursing. It would be nice to get your breast milk tested to see if the dose of medication your are taking is actually getting into your milk, however, you are unlikely to find a laboratory that can perform that kind of analysis. Drug levels in breast milk are of little interest to diagnostic laboratories and even many pharmaceutical companies aren't equipped for the process. However, it wouldn't hurt to ask your physician to make one or two calls to the company that developed the medication you are taking.

If you have exhausted all the alternatives, you are left with no other choice than to wean your baby. It will be a sad few days, but it isn't the end of the world. You need to be healthy if you are going to be a successful mother. Your baby will understand.

Remember that herbs are drugs, too! If you have become accustomed to using herbal remedies as supplements to or in replacement of traditional medications, be careful! While there is some scanty research about prescription medication and breast milk, there is virtually no data available regarding the safety of herbals for nursing mothers. Do not assume that just because a substance is obtained from a plant it is harmless. Nor should you conclude that just because you have taken an herbal medication without ill effect in the past it is safe to take while you are breastfeeding. Homeopathic remedies are usually so diluted that they are harmless (and usually ineffective), but before you take any medication, natural or chemically derived, consult your physician.

Appendix 3.

Nursing Your Premature Infant

You have already heard that breastmilk is clearly the best first food for newborns, but for premature infants the advantages are significantly greater. Their precarious situation and special vulnerabilities often require optimal nutrition for survival. If you deliver a premature baby, the milk that you produce will be uniquely suited to the needs of your immature infant in many ways that we understand and even more that we don't. For example, your milk will have a higher protein content and will contain a substance that encourages the absorption of vitamin D. It will also provide your preemie with several substances that offer increased immune protection and others that may provide protection against lung damage. Because premature infants are born before their nervous system is fully developed, the unique fat composition of breast milk is thought to play an even more important role in brain development than it does in term infants.

The bottom line is that regardless how long you were planning on nursing, I urge you in the strongest terms to provide your premature baby breast milk at least in the beginning. Most Newborn Intensive Care Units (NICUs) will take the initiative and introduce you to a lactation consultant or nurse educator who will help you begin the process of pumping and collecting your breast milk. Initially your preemie may be in such a precarious condition that the NICU staff forgets to get you involved in providing the nutritional support that your baby will need in a week or two. While breast milk may not be on the nursery staff's priority list for the first day or two, don't be afraid to speak up and ask what you can do to get the process started.

Having a sick child can be very frustrating because you would like to do something but you lack the medical expertise to help. Pumping and saving your milk is one of the few things that you can do that can make a real difference. Make sure that you have a good electrical pump. Save and freeze everything you can pump and carefully label it with date, time, and your baby's name. The NICU staff may provide you with containers. They may also ask you to submit a sample of your breast milk that they can culture for bacterial contamination. Even though your breast milk is full of all kinds of good stuff, it may actually make your baby sicker if it contains harmful bacteria. If the hospital laboratory detects unsafe levels of bacteria in the sample you give them, the nursing staff can help you to improve your technique in pumping and storing so that contamination can be minimized. The NICU staff will also want to know what, if any, medication you are taking to make sure that your milk is safe for your premature infant.

Depending on the severity and nature of your baby's problems, there may be a delay of several days or several weeks before the NICU staff will be able to use your breast milk. Don't be discouraged. Keep pumping. Once your baby starts growing rapidly, you may find that you will be happy to have banked all you did while you were waiting for your baby to improve.

The NICU staff may initially use a feeding tube passed into the baby's stomach to give him the breast milk you have supplied. If he is strong enough to take a nipple, ask if it is safe to offer him your breast. Even if your nipple seems too big for your preemie's mouth, try it anyway. Some studies have shown that skin-to-skin contact can help premature babies recuperate more quickly. The nurses can help you adjust your tiny baby without dislodging his various tubes and wires. If they think his condition is too precarious, they will tell you, but it never hurts to ask.

The lactation consultant may suggest that you use a "supplementer," which is sometimes known as a kangaroo pack. These systems consist of a plastic bag that holds your milk (or formula) and a thin, soft plastic tube that can be taped to your breast. While your baby is learning to suck on your nipple, the milk drips from the bag, through the tube and into his mouth. This not only allows him to be nourished while he is learning to suck on your nipple, but also rewards him for his efforts.

If your baby was extremely premature or is having trouble gaining weight, his doctors may add a nutritional fortifier to your breast milk for a week or so. This doesn't mean your milk is inferior. It merely means that your child's GI system is so immature that he must be offered extra calories until he turns the corner nutritionally. If you are having trouble pumping enough to keep your baby gaining, the NICU staff will offer formula when they have run out of the supply of your breast milk.

It is not unusual for a premature baby to go home from the hospital getting the bulk of his nutrition from a bottle. The nurses may have suggested that you offer him your breast only every third or every other feeding because nursing is more tiring for him. The transition to all breast feedings can take time. Work closely with your pediatrician as you decide exactly how quickly to make this shift. As your preemie gets bigger and stronger, you may have to get a little ugly with him if he still prefers the bottle. But, make sure the doctor thinks it is safe to "starve" him a little to encourage him to take your nipple.

INDEX

breastfeeding (*cont.*)
  in history, 2–3, 28–31
  during illnesses, 195–96
  interruptions of, 90, 106,
    125–26, 167–68
  need for fresh perspective on,
    1–2, 4–6
  popular and realistic scenario
    for, 37–38
  positions for, 82–85, 90–91,
    102, 109, 132
  in public, 10, 20–22, 59, 65,
    154, 161–62, 168–70
  realistic goals for, 42–43, 208–9
  reasons for, 9–17
  of second children, 2, 201–7
  statistics on, 1–3, 10, 17, 34,
    54, 64
breast milk, 11–16
  decreases in production of, 36,
    40–41
  efficient transfer of, 87–88
  immunological and anti-
    inflammatory properties of,
    12–13, 17, 33–34, 160, 216
  knowing when it is in, 118–19
  let-downs of, 24, 45, 119–20,
    122–27, 131–32, 155, 159
  nutritional value of, 11–12, 14,
    16, 18–19, 30–33, 125, 133,
    156–57, 186–87, 216–17
  physical appearance of, 48, 118,
    125
  pumping and storage of, 35–37,
    43, 47, 62–63, 65–67, 69,
    76, 86, 103–4, 106, 108,
    117–19, 121–22, 126–28,
    134, 139–40, 146, 149,
    153–55, 158, 161, 167–68,
    170, 172–77, 179–82, 184,
    196–97, 214, 216–17
  taste of, 158, 167, 170
  waiting for it to come in,
    113–21

breast pumps, 88–89, 108, 155
  purchasing of, 69–70, 76, 174
  strategies for use of, 174–75
breasts, 16, 120
  engorgement of, 8, 69, 88, 95,
    108, 115, 120–22, 184
  leaking of, 23–24, 40, 118–20,
    131, 155
  sizes of, 40, 90
breast shells, 88–89
breathing, 90–91, 96–98, 138
brick dust, 114–15, 118
burping, 124
  fatigue and, 137, 141
  husband's breastfeeding role
    and, 73–74
  pacifiers and, 144, 146
  technique for, 210–11

calcium, 16, 117, 141
chaos, 163–65, 204
CIGNA, 63
cleaning, 78, 116, 136, 181, 204–5
cold compresses, 121
colds, 158, 188, 195, 212–13
colic, 31, 140–41, 145–47
colostrum, 12, 103, 118
  on D-Day, 89–90
  on first day and night, 99,
    101
constipation, 125, 186–88, 194
continuous feeding, 30–31
cooking, 78, 181, 203–5
Coping with a Picky Eater
  (Wilkoff), 192
couplet nursing, 97
cow's milk, 11, 117, 141
  in formulas, 133, 187–88
  in months four through twelve,
    194, 197–98
cradle position, 83–84
cramps, 101, 151, 187
cribs, 68, 111, 137, 144, 163, 166,
    168

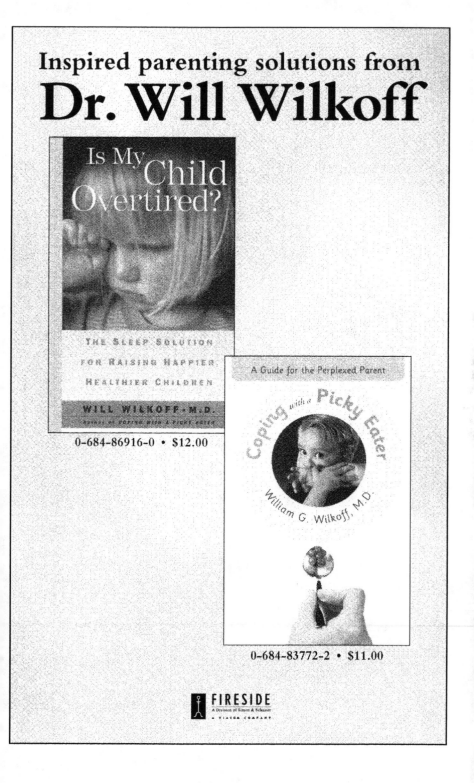